Praise for *Sex and the Perfect Lover*

"Offering a philosophical approach to sexual pleasure, the author draws upon Eastern teachings but uses a writing style and terminology more accessible to a Western audience. More than a simple sex manual, this slim volume condenses vast amounts of information into short, practical techniques for integrating mental and physical energies."

—*Library Journal*

"Taking from the ancient books of the Kama Sutra and the Tao, Iam's self-help guide to lovemaking will make you and your mate the perfect yin and yang combo."

—*Latina* magazine

"*Sex and the Perfect Lover* is not just a list of interesting sex positions. Rituals, massages, aphrodisiacs, and all sorts of strategies to take pleasure to unknown heights are included in this book."

—*el Nuevo Herald* (Miami)

"The reader will find several clues and tips for finding the perfect lover that we are all after."

—*El Diario–La Prensa* (New York)

Mabel Iam

ATRIA BOOKS

NEW YORK   LONDON   TORONTO   SYDNEY

SEX AND THE PERFECT LOVER

Tao,

Tantra,

and the

Kama Sutra

1230 Avenue of the Americas
New York, NY 10020

The Library of Congress has cataloged the hardcover edition as follows:

Iam, Mabel.
    [Amante perfecto. English]
    Sex and the perfect lover : tao, tantra, and the Kama sutra / Mabel Iam.
    p. cm.
    Includes bibliographical references.
          1. Sex—Religious aspects—Taoism. 2. Sex—Religious aspects—Tantrism.
    3. Sex instruction—Religious aspects—Taoism. 4. Sex instruction—Religious
    aspects—Tantrism. 5. Taoism. 6. Tantrism. I. Title.

    HQ61.I1613 2005
    306.7—dc22   2005053039

ISBN-13: 978-0-7432-8799-9
ISBN-10:   0-7432-8799-1
ISBN-13: 978-0-7432-9209-2 (Pbk)
ISBN-10:   0-7432-9209-X (Pbk)

This Atria Books trade paperback edition October 2006

10 9 8 7 6 5 4 3 2 1

ATRIA BOOKS is a trademark of Simon & Schuster, Inc.

Manufactured in the United States of America

For information about special discounts for bulk purchases,
please contact Simon & Schuster Special Sales:
1-800-456-6798 or business@simonandschuster.com.

If you want to write to the author,
please visit her website at www.mabeliam.com.

CONTENTS

ACKNOWLEDGMENTS

To my husband, Greg, the love of my life. He makes all my womanly fantasies come true. He inspires me and helps me grow each day with happiness and compassion. A great companion, a better friend, and the perfect lover.

With special love, to my beloved nephew and nieces, Ezequiel, Manuela, and Caterina, who are a part of my heart.

To the spiritual masters who taught me how to awaken my inner self and expand my awareness, especially Master Meishu Sama.

I would like to thank Judith Curr for her confidence in me, and, especially, Johanna Castillo for her friendship, love, and support of this new version of my beloved book.

I dedicate this book to women and men. May it enable them, on this very day, to make the commitment and the final decision to learn to be loved, without conflicts and in total freedom. By sharing this text, it is my humble intent for love in all of its perfection to become part of our lives and bestow on us its powerful blessing.

PROLOGUE

Whoever exalts Life knows nothing about Life—
that is why he has Life.
Whoever does not exalt Life seeks not to lose his Life—
that is why he has no Life.
Whoever exalts Life does not act nor does he have a purpose.
Whoever does not exalt Life does act and does have a purpose.
Whoever exalts Love acts but does not have a purpose.
Whoever exalts Justice does act and does have a purpose.
Whoever exalts rituals does act, and when someone does not reply,
he gestures with his arms and attracts him.
That is why: once the Tao is lost, there remains Life.
Once Life is lost, there remains Love.
Once Love is lost, there remains Justice.
Once Justice is lost, there remains Ritual.
Ritual is loyal, believing, weak, and the beginning of confusion.
Previous knowledge is the glitter of the Tao
and the beginning of foolishness.
That is why the upright man remains honest and is not found
among the weak.
He lives in the Being and not in the glitter.
He rejects that and takes this.

—Tao Te King, 38

INTRODUCTION

A man and a woman . . .
The man is the eagle that flies.
The woman is the nightingale that sings.
To fly is to master space.
To sing is to conquer the soul.
The man is a Temple.
The woman is the Altar.
Before the temple we uncover ourselves;
before the altar we kneel down . . .
The man is where the Earth ends.
The woman where Heaven starts.
—Victor Hugo

Sex and the Perfect Lover takes you by the hand on the road to experience pleasure and ecstasy on a permanent basis.

So you can travel that path and understand the meaning of true love. You can attain higher clarity of mind and understanding. The purpose of this book is to initiate you in the mastery of love and the enlightenment of your heart.

Each step down this road opens a door to deeper levels in yourself. You must go through three stages.

The first stage to be transcended is the one that involves Preparing for Love.

Once you have practiced all the techniques, once you have become versed in the arts of perfect love, you can continue on the way of the

Tao to a deeper inner level and arrive at a new stage—the Realization of Love.

To develop at this new stage, you have all the tools necessary in each of the chapters headed by these affirmations.

Once you have known the Realization of Love, you'll be able to Expand Love, because your heart is now ready to enlighten and glow with the eternal flame that dwells inside you.

The answers, the techniques, the visualizations, and the elements that will help you at each step are available in the affirmations presented in this chapter.

And since the Tao of Love is infinite, it has no end.
Or goals.
It is the eternal present.
When the three stages are reached,
the whole road has been covered.
The tao of love is always expanding,
that is why
it is immortal.
Here and now,
beyond sex,
you can love with your soul,
you already have the techniques
that lead you to be a perfect lover.

1

PREPARING

FOR LOVE

The heavens, as a result of the One, turned clear.
The earth, as a result of the One, became firm.

—Tao Te King, 39

1

THE PLEASURE OF THE TAO AND THE POLARITY OF SEX

The Tao: The Yin and Yang of Sex

When a woman unites with her man in love, all the magical power of the universe becomes integrated with this act, which then produces miracles both in heaven and on earth.

The Union of the Feminine with the Masculine

Even though it is impossible to know the precise origin of Taoist philosophy, it is known that around the year 500 B.C., Chinese scholar Lao-Tse researched and compiled its basic principles into a book that we know today as *Tao Te King.*

Just as the purpose of the Tao is to learn the supreme way to the self-actualization of a human being, the purpose of the Tao of a couple is to integrate love with sex and unite the male and female energies.

Representation of the Tao

The Tao is the unity of two principles: yin and yang. The symbol of yin and yang is a circle divided into two halves by an S-shaped line, with one half black and the other half white.

The circle represents the unity of the universe, consisting of the yin (black) aspects and the yang (white) aspects, inseparable in every manifestation of the whole. Within each half there is a smaller circle of the opposite color, which means that each principle contains the seed of the other. At the culminating moment of deployment and expression, each principle changes into its polar opposite so that the force of eternal equilibrium can do its work.

The Equilibrium of the Universe Depends on Polarity

According to the Tao, the universe is the product of the polarity existing within the primordial unity: rest and motion, contraction and expansion, condensation and scattering, moving backward and moving forward. From the most simple and peculiar manifestations to the most complex and universal ones, every being expresses this original polarity. The interrelationship between yin and yang generates all living things that inhabit the universe.

The Tao philosophy is based on the search for balance and the integration of opposing energy forces that are complementary to each other.

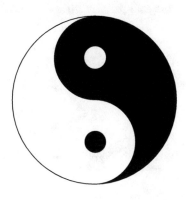

THE YIN AND YANG SYMBOL

Yin and Yang

Yin energy represents the feminine: passivity, night, wetness, cold, water, and the moon. The woman, with all her sexual secretions and fluids, constitutes a yin essence that provides the necessary protection that allows the male's semen to become an embryo.

The woman contains an inexhaustible reserve of yin energy that is activated by sexual arousal. The female orgasm strengthens vital energy, improves health, and prolongs youth.

Due to the fact that a woman's sexual potential is more energetic and open, almost all texts on this subject place a greater emphasis on educating the man so both lovers can reach an equivalent level of satisfaction.

Yang energy represents the masculine: activity, day, dryness, sun, and fire. Man's sperm is a precious gift, the source of his physical health and vital energy. This vital energy will diminish unless it is compensated by an equivalent amount of female yin energy, which is why the man must seek to satisfy the woman each time he has sexual contact with her. That way, both will benefit the other during each act of lovemaking: he will strengthen his vital essence, and she will stimulate and intensify her yin essence.

According to Taoist thinking, the sexual feature of yin is slower excitation, but this also means that a woman is slower to quit at the moment when she needs more sexual stimulation. On the contrary, yang's sexual feature is easy excitability, which allows the man to achieve maximum pleasure instantly.

The man needs to learn to prolong the sexual act without reaching orgasm so that both energies can merge and fuse. By increasing the time his member remains inside the woman, he will absorb the yin essence that will in turn revitalize him.

When the man's yang force and the woman's yin force unite, they create life in the universe.

Infinite Pleasure

There are physical and mental exercises that enable a couple having sexual problems to find a balance. These ancient techniques are very effective for people who play routine, stereotyped, or rigid roles in their sexual relations, which may eventually lead to a loss of sexual desire.

First of all, lovers should work on developing the tenderness of their feelings and express them through caressing each other. Each partner must caress the other in a slow and soft manner, with yin sensitivity. In doing so, not only do the mouth and the fingers take part, but so does the whole body, including those parts that are not usually explored erotically.

While the partners caress each other, both should focus mentally on the image of a sun embracing the moon with its light beams—two vital energies becoming integrated.

The man should excite the woman until they both reach maximum wetness in their erogenous zones. Upon achieving this yin sensation, it is time for the intervention of the yang, with the man's penetration of the woman until the couple achieves maximum pleasure.

Having completed the sexual act in a state of ecstasy, the couple must wait a few minutes and allow their bodies to relax completely. When they reach this restful state, the lovers should visualize the image of an integrated earth and sky, while holding hands and kissing at the same time.

If the lovers start caressing each other again, they may get excited anew and perform the sexual act more than twice a day.

If a couple performs these exercises every day for some time, they will successfully harmonize their yin and yang energies and will experience the highest embodiment of love.

2

THE SUPREME WAY: THE TAO OF SPIRITUAL EVOLUTION THROUGH TANTRA

Tantra: Another Way to Sacred Pleasure

The art of the bedroom constitutes the climax
of human emotions
and includes the Supreme Way.

—Vishvasara Tantra

The word *tantra* comes from the union of the root word *tan*, meaning "to extend, to expand," and the suffix *tra,* referring to an instrument. *Tantra,* therefore, is an instrument for the expansion of ordinary consciousness in order to access the root of the self as well as the unknown potential that it may be possible to use and awaken.

The Tantra discipline, or Tantra yoga, was developed through the rituals, practices, and meditations found in various sacred books from

India. These books, which are over two thousand years old, were written as dialogues between the Hindu god Shiva, "the penetrating power of focused energy," and his mate Shakti, who represents the creative female force, sometimes called "the power of Tantra." In Tantra, the universe is alive. From the most distant star to the smallest subatomic particle, everything is inhabited by some form of consciousness. The universe is consciousness and energy combined. In practice, this leads to a respect for all life, both animal and vegetable. When anyone harms any form of life, they are damaging their own life—ecology becomes cosmic.

For couples seeking a significantly different way to relate to each other and keep love and passion alive for a long time, Tantra provides some very important tools.

Tantric sex does not promise instant results—it is not a "one-minute" technique to gain sexual skills. But for couples who wish to enrich their relationship, it can release a special type of energy that enhances harmony and increases sexual pleasure and intimacy. Tantric sex can create an extraordinary sense of companionship between the partners.

Tantra's Ancient Secrets

The mysterious and often misrepresented Tantra discipline includes a set of ancient techniques, doctrines, and rituals designed to unite the human mind with the infinite. According to Tantra, the universe was born from the cosmic union of the male and female principles. This conception includes Tantric sex, combining the wisdom of the pleasures inherent in human nature and the pleasures that come to us through the mystical path that bridges human love to divine love.

Tantric Sexuality

Tantra seeks the expansion of the mind by freeing energy from the fetters that bind it to the dense dimensions of matter. Tantra is the system whereby Shakti, the primordial energy, is released. To achieve this, it is necessary to work diligently with a proper diet, proper breathing (pranayama), proper exercise, proper relaxation, and proper thoughts (meditation).

At the same time, making love is an ideal opportunity for the conscious circulation of energy, and either partner may cause his or her own energy as well as the energy of the partner to circulate.

Energy circulates when we make love, but it is often lost due to a lack of awareness. It is important to familiarize ourselves with the sensation of a free flow of energy in order to recognize it consciously. It is surprising to realize how easily the mind is able to feel the flow of energy if we let our intuition get in contact with the body of our partner. Deep breathing enables us to experience the energy flow. We can see that certain parts of the body feel awakened, while others are asleep or less stimulated.

Tantric erotic positions, known as bandhas (locks), were devised to inwardly channel the energy flowing outward. Hands and feet are used frequently as aids in this extremely important process: to cause sexual energy to circulate instead of that energy being lost. An essential ingredient in Tantric practice is to honor the inner spirit. That is how love assumes its liberating and truly eternal character.

The sexual relationship consists then of delivering one's sexuality to another person. When someone accepts the sexual act as a gift, exchanges take place at various levels: a physical exchange of secretions, a psychophysical exchange of vital polarities and energies, a karmic exchange through the convergence of destinies, and a spiritual exchange in the communion of spirits. All these exchanges enhance the quality of the couple's relationship.

Tantra does not advise prolonged sexual abstinence, since it leads to the accumulation of unnatural sexual currents inside the body. Retention consists of maintaining pleasure as a light in the midst of a storm. Tantric texts underscore the importance of "absorbing your partner's equivalent" when there is a release of vital fluids. The loss of semen, which originates from all parts of the body, weakens the man and shortens his life. To counteract the loss caused by ejaculation, the man must consciously absorb the woman's secretions, for which there are various techniques.

In any event, the retention of semen or the conscious control of ejaculation is a personal issue, since it doesn't affect a twenty-year-old young man in the same way as a fifty-year-old adult. The loss of energy through ejaculation has a different meaning for each individual, so each must decide when and how to establish his own frequency.

At the highest levels of eroticism, orgasm becomes merely a point in time, a further incentive in the state of intense and continuous physical and emotional splendor that lovers successfully evoke in each other. Sex is not considered a sensation, but a feeling. The attraction is not an appetite, but an "eye-to-eye contact." Love is not a reaction, but a carefully fostered creation, a prolonged mental and bodily ecstasy whose flames are kept alive by the prolonged stimulation of the sexual organs and not by the mere reciprocal release. In this sense, the rituals accompanying the sex acts also convey charges of accumulated energy.

The positions and internal contractions that take place in the course of the Tantric union are based on this conception of sexual love. But the special condition of inner splendor that they provoke only manifests when the erotic focus of attention shifts from the external and sensorial personification of desire to the inner goddess of which all external women are a manifestation. In this sense, the satisfaction of the woman is extremely important, since only with such satisfaction will a woman bestow all of her initiation potential on her lover. Both the woman and man, therefore, are key to reciprocal delight. This does not mean that one will lose value in the eyes of the other. Quite the contrary—because each will become a divinity in the other person's eyes.

3

INNER DIVINITY, SELF-KNOWLEDGE, AND THE PATH OF THE TAO

The Road to Perfection

Sex is not only an act whereby bodies find each other with a greater or lesser degree of surrender and satisfaction. It isn't a dirty word either. It is the starting point of life. We need to become friends with the powerful sexual energy that modifies all things.

Oftentimes we behave as if body and sex were our enemies. The perception of our sexuality, whether complete, normal, or unexplored, is a true reflection of our lives.

When well understood, sexuality holds the key that opens the door to the knowledge of being and our inner self. It doesn't matter if we still have issues pending on this subject; we always have the opportunity to achieve deep knowledge on how to develop our sexual energy through various physical exercises, seeking out those that best fit our lifestyle and personality and are compatible with the people with whom we relate sexually and emotionally. When the body and the spirit are in balance, you start the journey to total and complete love.

Tantra's Erotic Rituals

We can develop our sexual energy alone or as a couple through various techniques: active meditations, visualizations, rituals, and through the knowledge of various symbols, such as internal colors and energy centers, or chakras.

This attitude endows the relationship with many advantages. We grow closer to our beloved with the respect and devotion he or she deserves, and by so doing, we evoke in him or her, and therefore in ourselves, a higher dimension. Every human weakness we see on a daily basis in the other person disappears, at least during this sacred and devotional act we perform. The love relationship turns into mutual stimulation for the awakening of consciousness.

When lovers manage to reserve a space to see each other and themselves as higher beings, a type of energy is created that is quite helpful in their daily life together.

Sexual energy is increased when stimulated by the erotic ritual. This is the basis for the process of Tantric transformation.

Sacred Space and Body

Partners who have been living together for a long time usually place too much emphasis on the human defects of the other partner. Even when they love each other, if they have partially lost their passion, they must arrive at the mutual decision to understand each other and feel again the intensity of the first period of their relationship. The force of sexual ritual helps them achieve this.

The first thing a couple needs to do is to enter a sacred space-time, which is a lot more important than simply setting aside time and having a bedroom with flowers and decorations. It also entails entering a unique space-time—an inner place where there is no past or future, a place where everything converges. This magic place is created in the mind, in the awareness that something extraordinary is going to take place.

Explained in simpler terms, it is like entering a space where a ritual will be held, while remaining aware that we are passing into a magic place where the here and now prevail—where we have left behind our problems and concerns and any memory of the past.

In this space we'll approach the body of our lover as we would sacred soil. The body must be washed, purified, and perfumed in acknowledgment of its beauty and its transcendental dimension. Both bodies and both lovers are the expression of divinity. By loving each other, they rejoice in life, and energy is awakened.

4

THE GODDESS
AND THE PATH TO THE HEART

Awaken Pleasure in the Goddess and You Will Be Able to Kindle Her Heart

*"There is no way to open up
other than the female way.
There is no yesterday or now or tomorrow,
or any other fortune but woman, nor any other kingdom,
pilgrimage or yoga,
or prayer, or magic formula,
or any other fulfillment than what woman provides."*

—Shaktisangama, Tantra: Beyond the Orgasm

Awakening the Goddess

The act of lovemaking is an experience beyond comparison, both in regard to the sensations and to the feelings that reveal our deepest, remotest core. This experience is intimately related to erotic play. The internal female energy has the role of initiating this game, while the male energy has the function of exciting and provoking the sexual impulse.

In direct contrast to animals, human beings display eroticism and are able to dissociate sexual expression from the instinct to procreate. Going a step further, followers of Tantra believe in the possibility and freedom to choose the moment of pleasure.

Sexual dissatisfaction arises in a couple, for starters, because the first orgasm is only the beginning for a woman, while ejaculation ends the man's erection and interrupts female excitation. These differences confirm the fact that a woman needs sexual stimulation beyond the genital aspect, since the first orgasm is not enough to truly satisfy her.

The question is, then, what can be done so that the woman's enjoyment continues beyond the first orgasm?

The Poles of Limitless Pleasure

The woman has two sensitive poles loaded with sexual energy. In Tantric philosophy, the North Pole is the clitoris, the most accessible spot and so far the only one recognized. The South Pole is deeper and is called the Sacred Spot. Some sexual therapists refer to it as the mysterious G-spot.

The clitoris sits like a bell on the upper part of the vulva. It's the only organ in the body whose function is to generate pleasure. Even though the head of the clitoris is small, most women are able to touch and stimulate it easily. She can also stimulate it with the male organ as foreplay to penetration.

But finding the Sacred Spot requires such a sense of touch that it is difficult for a woman to find it by herself. If you find this Sacred Spot, you will be able to liberate the womanly sexual and spiritual potential, which then acts as a healing power.

Some women have been able to locate this spot by themselves, by pressing two fingers inside the vagina upward toward the navel while simultaneously pressing down with the other hand just above the pubic bone. If a woman succeeds in stimulating or massaging this area, the spot will swell and may become palpable to her partner. However, for most women this part of the process of awakening requires the gentle touch of their partner, who must be ready to respect the physically and psychologically vulnerable nature of this site. That is why Tantric discipline provides methods to assimilate rapidly the knowledge about female pleasure and the poles of ecstasy.

The Sacred Spot, as known by Tantra followers, is located deep in the vagina and is much more protected than the clitoris. Finding it and stimulating it produces the most intense pleasure that can be experienced, but to achieve this, a couple needs much patience and dedication.

If the woman hasn't had positive sexual experiences, this area must be caressed most carefully and gently. Little by little, the couple will learn to stimulate it and this will bring about a physical and spiritual well-being in the woman that transcends the sexual aspects. It is most important for the couple to overcome their prejudices and learn how to kindle the inner flame that sustains the spirit dwelling in each of us. This way, lovers will be able to purify their negative experiences.

A woman must know her body and explore her satisfaction without guilt, so that she is able to tell her lover what she really needs. Having a full relationship increases self-esteem and creates a sense of vitality and enthusiasm.

The Goddess' Pleasure

Tantra places a primordial importance on love and sexuality. The performance is a sacred ritual that seeks to connect one's physical and spiritual energy. This translates into the names given to the organs: *lingam* for the male organ, which means "shaft of light," and *yoni* for the female organs, which translates as "sacred space."

In Tantra, spiritual consciousness is intimately related to the awakening of the goddess, who holds the power of universal creative energy. The power possessed by female energy is so great that at times it becomes uncontrollable. That is why Tantra seeks, in the sexual act, the pleasure of the woman as a form of ecstasy and as a form of evolution for both partners.

In order to achieve this supreme pleasure, the woman's Sacred Spot must be found, but this requires patience and experience. Learning to know ourselves can provide us with multiple satisfactions, both sexually and in life in general, but few women know their true intensity because sex was, for centuries, a taboo subject. Many men and women still experience sex with a certain degree of guilt or disrespect. Maybe this is why most couples don't know or don't share their needs, which prevents them from understanding each other.

Many people are not aware of the ways of pleasure and tend to believe that sexual stimulation is all in plain sight. But if the woman is successful in her search for her Sacred Spot, she will be able to experience explosive orgasms. This uncontrollable sensation, and the transforming power it entails, can even provoke a certain degree of fear if the woman is not ready to experience such a high degree of intensity.

Perhaps not being able to manage their most primary instincts has led women to repress them, and men to be afraid of not being able to control such an overwhelming force. We need to stimulate and motivate each other in order to awaken the dormant energy hidden in our bodies, so that we can get in touch with the very energy of the universe.

The power of pleasure is already inside of you—you only have to decide to become aware of your divine possibilities.

5

SACRED SPACE AND MEDITATION TECHNIQUES

Meditation with Sexual Impulse

When we say the word *meditation,* the image that usually comes to mind is that of a guru or master yogi sitting motionless for his entire life. Nothing could be further from the truth: there are meditation techniques that are static, but there are others that are performed while we are in motion.

What can meditation do for us? First of all, it is a tool for self-knowledge and an instrument for relaxation. It can help us focus our energies on the here and now, on the present moment, on the space-time we set aside for sacred love.

In short, meditation is a tool to become even more connected to the sacred dimensions of ecstasy.

A Meditation Practice

The most simple and classic method of becoming initiated in the practice of meditation is learning how to relax and concentrate on one's breathing. Let's explore the following practice.

Sit comfortably, with your back upright. Your hands should rest on your legs, close to your knees, or both on your lap, palms facing upward, the left hand beneath the right hand. Your shoulders should be relaxed, without unnecessary tension in the face or neck.

Breathe in by raising your shoulders a little and let them drop as you exhale. Repeat this three or four times. You'll see how, when you open your chest to breathe, you feel it expand.

Then carefully observe whether the air slightly brushes your lips and whether your nostrils open and close a little when breathing in and out.

Focus on the air entering through the right nostril, and notice if the air temperature is different from that of the air entering through the left nostril.

Does the air have color? What color does it suggest? The air entering through the right nostril—what color does it suggest to you? And how about the air entering through the left nostril? Where does the air go?

We always use our eyes to see what lies outside—but now we're looking in. We see how the air goes down little by little—is it dense or subtle? Is it like a warm light that fills the lungs little by little, or is it like a bolt of lightning that flashes?

Become aware that when air fills your whole chest, you feel happy. You perceive that there is life inside of you. When you're calm, warm air relaxes and expands your chest.

The most important thing is to remain in the quiet of your inner self, observing what happens inside and outside of you, as a witness to all.

Full Breathing

Full breathing consists of working both your lungs and your entire abdomen to achieve correct deep respiration.

To learn how to breathe correctly, it is helpful to lie down on a mattress on the floor. The mattress you use should not be too soft. Make sure you will not be interrupted for the next fifteen to twenty minutes.

Pay attention to your thoughts and let them pass as if they were clouds—do not identify with any of them. After a few minutes of relaxation, place one hand on your abdomen and the other on your chest, and softly breathe out all the air through your nose, emptying your lungs completely.

Try to keep your lungs empty for a few seconds and then breathe in slowly, inflating only your abdomen until you have filled up the lower portion of the lungs completely. Without making any effort, you'll feel how the diaphragm expands downward to allow the lower and middle portions of your lungs to fill with air.

When breathing out, take advantage of that moment and empty your mind of all thoughts—imagine that your daily tensions and emotions are also being released. Contract your abdomen and continue expelling the air little by little.

Repeat this process for a minimum of ten minutes.

With your mind emptied of worries and concerns and your body revitalized by the intake of fresh oxygen, you'll be in better condition to focus your attention on the here and now of sacred sex.

6

THE POWER OF THOUGHT
IN THE TAO OF SEXUAL MAGIC

The Depths of Pleasure

When you leave all doubts behind, you'll be able to expand and see your soul devoid of emotion. The smiling gods will line the sides of the road to bid you welcome. When you touch heaven with your hands and your heart flows over the earth, your whole existence will have true meaning.

To develop sexual energy, we have already talked about the following techniques:

Relaxation
Deep breathing
Meditation

Another practice that is both effective and helpful is erotic visualization. In addition, you can learn to develop the capacity to focus your energy on your heart.

Erotic Visualization

In a state of relaxation, in almost meditative awareness, start to visualize your lover's body with your mind's eye. Imagine it in as much detail as possible.

Then imagine how you could give it pleasure, what erogenous zones you should stimulate, and how you want to do it so your lover can achieve a total state of ecstasy.

Take a few moments to visualize calmly and in detail each step you want to take to satisfy your lover, how your lover's body reacts, and how ecstasy is being achieved.

You'll notice that a state of inner connection ensues that makes you feel extremely excited. You'll feel a deep desire to embrace your partner and perform the sexual act as quickly as possible. But if you do so, all the stimulation and prior exercising will be lost.

For a man, the most important thing is to control ejaculation and share the magic of sexual energy in an ever more prolonged fashion with his partner.

The Heart's Flame

While maintaining sexual contact and prolonged ecstasy, focus your awareness on the awakening of energy in the center of your heart, a very powerful energy.

Three extremely important spiritual rays are concentrated in the heart, consisting of different luminosities:

1. Pink light, which is directly related to unconditional love.
2. Blue light, which is related to the power of creation.
3. Yellow light, which represents the totality of the self.

A Ritual of Love, Power, and Wisdom

Continue in a state of relaxation, naked in front of your partner. Start to visualize a flame that includes the three aforementioned colors in your heart. You'll notice that this triple flame shines light on your partner's heart as if it were a torch of fire.

You and your lover must perform this exercise simultaneously, visualizing the other wrapped in the three colors emanating from the heart. If imagining these colors turns out to be difficult, observe a flame together before performing the ritual and you'll both be able to see the three colors and the light they shine.

Then imagine the same fire or ardent heat coming out of the heart and being received by you and your lover. This way the union achieved will be stronger and more complete, before and during sexual contact.

7

ENERGY AND EROTIC MOTION

As a form of yoga within the Hindu tradition, Tantra emphasizes the importance of knowing how vital energy circulates within the body in order to harmonize the circulation of this energy and develop its power.

The body is energy in action, but in order to develop the power of this vital energy, we have to know the points where this energy is concentrated and distributed.

According to Oriental teaching, when these points, referred to as *chakras*, become blocked—whether due to stress, emotional problems, inhibitions, phobias, or fear of contact, among other things—a person's sexual vitality diminishes considerably.

What Are Chakras?

They are seven centers distributed along the length of the body, connected to the glands that regulate the normal functioning of the respective areas of the body. When these centers malfunction, we are more susceptible to contracting various diseases that also affect our behavior and emotions.

Meditation and visualization help unblock these centers and harmonize their functions. The center corresponding to sexual energy is the one that is most often blocked.

How to Unblock the Sexuality Center

We can unblock our sexual energy by means of localization, relaxation, and motion. The more we relax and are aware of our emotional and sexual flow, the better we'll be able to control our personal power and enjoy our intimate relationships. Moving the areas of the body where sexual energy flows in a smooth and harmonious fashion helps us get to know that energy and enjoy it.

How to Enjoy the Erotic Rhythm

The rhythm of pleasure became intertwined between
our legs to the rhythm of our hips.
The whole night we merged
in an erotic dance as though in a ritual.
The sweet friction of love's energy made us
shine in the darkness.
To our surprise, we discovered the sunrise
while we reflected our own light as if it were the moon.

The purpose of these techniques is to respect, deepen, and stimulate the natural rhythms of the body. Through various motions in a state of relaxation, we can control and increase vitality and at the same time prevent muscle fatigue.

An Exercise to Prepare the Sexual Rhythm

This exercise can be performed individually or as a couple. It is performed standing up and walking.

First, you must completely relax your body. Focus your attention on your flow of energy while combining the rhythms of respiration with slow motions that use the weight of the body to move your arms and legs in an arch-like motion.

Then, with your legs apart and slightly bent, make short movements to observe each muscle's reflex and connection to respiration and circulation. Also note each muscle's direct relation to other parts of the body that relax or contract to enable the motion.

Usually, expansion motions are accompanied by an inhalation, and contraction motions by an exhalation. The flow of motions must be continuous.

The objective is to achieve "harmony of body and spirit" by being attentive to respiration and the way energy circulates throughout the body.

Dance and Joy: Sexual Rhythms, Step by Step

Men and women have different tempos of sexual response. If you wish for a maximum love connection with your partner, you need to experience the different rhythms, which range from wild, erotic rhythms to the softest and most tender cadences. Your sensations must become tuned to those of your lover, until both of you reach sexual fulfillment.

The First Rhythm Is the Sexual Impulse

This rhythm is directly related to the mutual attraction between the two partners. It is characterized by the seduction each partner provokes in the other.

The Second Rhythm Is Excitation

This tempo is spontaneous and is usually expressed more slowly in the woman and more quickly in the man. It depends exclusively on the erotic game that was induced by the first rhythm. It is important to personalize your ardor to stimulate your lover's erogenous zones.

The Third Rhythm Is the Orgasmic Rhythm

This rhythm is the result of the previous ones. Just like in a dance, lovers preserve an erotic energy of both instinctive and emotional encounters. This stage concentrates the mystery of the ecstasy of sexual rhythm.

The Fourth Rhythm Is Consummation

At this level an infinite explosion is achieved that transcends the limits of physical satisfaction and awakens the lovers' indescribable feelings. This burst, this explosive ecstasy, can only be attained through mutual surrender, while following the rhythm of love. When each lover adapts to the sexual response of the partner, the sexual act does not end with the orgasm—quite the contrary; after the temporary release, these techniques rekindle sexual pleasure.

The Game of Mirrors

Lovers can perform the Game of Mirrors exercise, which will help them appreciate the sensations of their partner. This technique is geared to polish your perceptions, so you can better appreciate your lover as a pleasurable object.

1. Lovers exchange sexual roles, by mutual agreement. This exercise is based on imitating the motions that are naturally performed by your partner in the course of the erotic game. First, one partner performs the active role and then the other will imitate him or her. This mirroring technique is the same technique used to learn any dancing move.

2. The marvelous thing about human beings while making love is that they can acquire knowledge and learn from different experiences by getting in contact with creativity and pleasure. Astonishing results can be achieved by performing this exercise once a week and then once a month.

The couple that finds a unique rhythm transforms sexuality into the true art of loving.

8

EROTIC DANCE

Technique to Prepare
for the Erotic Dance

Preparing for the erotic dance takes approximately an hour and consists of four steps. It is important to play music that is strong and vibrant, but is without lyrics, in order to avoid mental associations and memories. The purpose of this exercise is to induce mental silence.

First Step

For ten to fifteen minutes, relax and allow your body to move or quiver. Free yourself from all inhibitions. Feel how energy ascends from your feet throughout all of your body.

Relax your head and allow it to move wherever you wish. This can be done with your eyes open or closed.

Second Step

For ten to fifteen minutes, dance spontaneously as if you were a child. Let your body lead you inside that spontaneous rhythm.

Third Step

Close your eyes and be still, whether sitting down or standing up. The important thing is to be aware of anything you feel inside your body, such as restlessness, calm, tingling, or excitation.

Fourth Step

Quietly and with your eyes closed, notice the flow of your vital energy after moving. Breathe ever more slowly until you feel complete ecstasy with this natural dance of your body.

If the dance is performed as a couple, lovers ideally should try to coordinate their rhythms. They can touch each other and, with their legs apart, softly move their hips in mutual rhythm.

9

THE EXPLOSIVE ORGASM

We have already explored various elements that are conducive to achieving an intense sexual and spiritual relationship. All of these elements are steps that help us get in tune with both our own rhythms and with those of our partner. The steps also lead to achieving an explosive orgasm.

Before achieving an explosive orgasm, it is very pleasurable to softly massage your partner with a moisturizing lotion or cream on the lower back, the spine, and the inside surface of the arms and legs.

In men, the central area of their feet is particularly sensitive. The liver, which controls and releases the additional blood needed for erection, benefits directly from this stimulation.

How to Achieve the Explosion

In order to achieve a balance, the man must take in the woman's fluids. Taoist sexual discipline teaches men the "Great Liberation of the Three Peaks." This means that the man must absorb the secretions of the woman's lips and tongue, breasts, and vagina, or mons veneris. The man must lick up these secretions because, according to Taoists, they are very healthy. The man should use his tongue to stimulate the woman's mouth, breasts, the upper part of her pelvis, and the inside of her vagina.

How to Recognize the Signs that Indicate Sexual Enjoyment in Women

Practitioners of the Tao of Love assert that it is possible to recognize the degree of female pleasure by discovering the "Five Signs." If a lover pays attention to each of them, he will know how to make the right move at the right time.

1. When the woman's face blushes and her body temperature rises, her partner should start to play tenderly.
2. The man should penetrate the woman when he observes that her nipples are hard and small drops of sweat appear around her nose.
3. If he notices dryness in her throat and lips, he should thrust more vigorously.
4. When female lubrication turns slippery, the man should achieve the deep explosion. He needs to keep moving his pelvis while penetration lasts and not stop. He should softly squeeze the woman's body against his, but each time with more insistence.
5. The last sign will be the secretion of a viscous fluid on the woman's thighs. This indicates that she has reached the high tide of orgasmic explosion. At this moment, the man should begin breathing exercises in order to withhold ejaculation for a longer time, which makes it possible to employ different positions in search of the supreme pleasure.

10

THE BODY AND ITS COLORS

The Tao of Sex and Its Colors

If you fill your life with the proper colors, you will be able to change your feelings and your perceptions and noticeably improve each sexual experience.

Sex and Colors

Sexual rituals have long been performed by using various supporting elements—from candles of different colors to special garments whose colors, textures, and styles varied depending on the ritual's origin.

Nothing escapes the power of the colors in a rainbow. In our daily lives, we usually spend considerable time choosing the colors we use to paint each room of our house, and we recognize the energy emitted by the colors of crystals and stones that shine in earrings or other jewels.

The discipline of chromotherapy studies the effects of colors on people. By using some of these findings, it is possible to reestablish the natural power of our energy centers by visualizing specific colors, or by using illumination, choosing colors that strengthen and reinforce our erogenous zones.

"Nothing is true or false—it all depends on the color of the glass you look through," says a Spanish proverb, and it contains more than a grain of truth. Colors are nothing but light beams reflected or emitted by the objects we see. This luminous radiation has the power to exert a healing influence through the various energy channels in our body.

Likewise, working internally and externally with colors modifies our disposition and the "waves" we emit.

The Purpose of Visualizing Each Color

Yellow

Yellow is a natural stimulant of emotions. It helps harmonize wishes and desires and make them come true.

Blue

Blue is a cold color that relieves anxiety and helps control attacks of obsessive sexual attraction.

White

White is used in purification rituals and is related to the cleanliness that should precede a sexual relation or a love union.

Navy Blue

Blue is a great spiritual generator. It magnetizes people's environments, thereby attracting states of peace, protection, and safety.

Gray

The neutral color par excellence, gray is useful for creating environments that foster an objective understanding of what's happening around us.

Brown

Brown is associated with the persistence and patience of those who help us grow spiritually.

Orange

Orange has a soothing effect that acts directly on the central nervous system and increases our attention span.

Black

Black absorbs light. It is associated with female energy and with the dark side of the Tao symbol, but its effect may vary depending on how it is used.

Red

Red symbolizes sexual power. It increases eroticism and provides strength and endurance. It fills the blood with oxygen and clears its toxins.

Pink

Pink preserves love in sexual relationships and fuses love and erotic passion into a bond.

Green

Green is associated with nature and living energy. Its hypnotic vibrations bring calm to the body and mind.

Violet

Violet is the manifestation of the spirit, which is why it is the color used to transform negative emotions and thoughts.

Multicolor Pleasure

When you think of two lovers, you never imagine them vibrating together in black and white. What color excites you?

Colors produce an energy vibration that acts on different planes, but the art of making love requires more than a mere game with colors. The culmination of pleasure is marked by a variety of colors felt only by those who are willing to experiment with the various hues.

Colors and Sexual Motivation

Colors express moods and emotions that are directly related to concrete psychic meanings. They also clearly exert a physiological effect. Whenever we have problems with our partner due to a lack of sexual desire or because there isn't a strong erotic chemistry, we can use different colors to increase pleasure to its utmost level.

The most common practice is to use colors as part of the environment's decor. For example, to foster moments of pleasure, you can place a specially colored light in the room. Red symbolizes passion, vitality, and strength. Orange is a source of refreshing energy and is useful in solving communication problems. It also enhances the physical connection. The use of various hues of red and other bright colors in lingerie accentuates the female form.

Visible Impact

We must be particularly aware of how we prepare ourselves for the ritual of passion—what clothes, makeup, or other enhancements we choose to wear before making love. Certain color combinations continue to exert a subliminal effect on our lover's mind after the moment of intimacy.

These colors cause the same magnetism as the colors that are used to control city traffic. They are colors that should stand out from our surroundings to increase our lover's focus on our body and the situation at hand. Here are some possible combinations:

Black and yellow
Green and white
Red and white
Blue and white

Incorporating any of these color combinations into the environment where the moment of intimacy is to take place will increase and enhance the visual impact. Start with the bed sheets and include any bodily accessories. When a couple is having problems, the first impact a change in the environment can have is to arouse interest, curiosity, and finally excitation.

The Inner Circle and Its Colors

A human being is a bundle of energies as vibrant as colors. If we have a positive relationship with our partner, an effective technique is to concentrate on a protective energy before beginning foreplay. Already in the nude, both partners can visualize each other wrapped in a spiral of a particular color, depending on the effect they wish to achieve.

11

VISUALIZING DIVINE PLEASURE

Sex can be happy,
but only love is a true delight.

Visualizing Divine Pleasure

You can use the infinite energy of this visualization to explore pleasure beyond its known limits.

First Step

Relax your body completely and keep breathing until you reach a state of complete serenity.

Second Step

Imagine a white light penetrating through your head.

Third Step

Visualize the body's energy centers, with their respective colors, as beams of light that open up and overcome whatever is blocked.

Fourth Step

Feel that each center is interconnected with the others, and finish the exercise with the pleasant sensation brought about by the harmony of each color.

If you practice this exercise for a few minutes every day, the change will be instantaneous and the general condition of your body will improve noticeably. You'll be able to observe a change in your relationship as a couple on the emotional and sexual planes.

When you awaken your internal energy, the expression of pleasure is complete and limitless.

12

HOW TO REACH
THE CORE OF ECSTASY

Making love is one of the healthiest and most beneficial exercises for the human body, since it requires exerting oneself as when practicing a sport, and therefore it has the same effects: it keeps the abdominal muscles in shape, increases lung capacity, and improves blood flow and hormone exchanges.

An erotic book from the Ming Dynasty taught that a man must penetrate a woman 1,200 times before reaching true satisfaction. Time-wise, this equals about forty minutes of actual sexual acts. From the point of view of physical exertion, this would keep anyone in pretty good shape.

Love contact and communication are vitally important for all human beings. The happiness and well-being produced by a sexual relationship are almost impossible to find in other activities. Caresses and tender words are instruments that bring about great benefits as part of a couple's interaction. The Tao of Love recommends the following:

1. Before making love, create an atmosphere that is conducive to intimacy.
2. Relax, empty your mind, and then focus only on caresses and stimulating words.
3. Leisurely stimulate your partner's sensitive areas and invite your partner to do likewise.
4. Change position every ten minutes.
5. The number of times a week you make love may vary, but there must be only one ejaculation in those seven days.

13

PREPARING FOR THE TRUE KAMA SUTRA

The True Meaning of the Kama Sutra

The Kama Sutra was written in India between the third and fifth centuries, and its authorship is attributed to the scholar Vatsyayana. It combines Taoist sexual techniques gathered from Chinese bedroom books with the seduction methods described by the Roman poet Ovid, although the Kama Sutra places more emphasis on love (distinguishing it from desire and passion) than did Ovid and the Chinese. Vatsyayana repeatedly interrupts his descriptions of sexual techniques or seduction to insist that the rules do not apply to people in love, who only have to let themselves go and be led by instinct.

Most people associate the Kama Sutra simply with multiple positions in which to perform the sexual act, a mixture of pornography and acrobatics. In the Orient, the true meaning of the Kama Sutra lies very far from this purely gymnastic idea.

From both the perspective of the Tao of Love and that of Tantra, every sexual union is sacred and reproduces the ultimate act of creation: the union of the male and female cosmic principles, a union that is the cause of the created and manifest universe. Sexual contact, no matter how trivial it may seem, is sacred and cosmic, even when those who experience such sexual contact are unaware of this.

The Kama Sutra teaches a series of *asanas*, which are yoga positions that have ritualistic meaning. Its purpose is to "divinize" the couple and their sexuality. Without this spiritual component, the Kama Sutra loses its ritualistic meaning.

The aim of the positions is not only to experience sensual voluptuousness but also to facilitate meditation as a couple. Some positions enable them to prolong the sexual union for up to two hours without the need to move much, so as not to disturb the internalization of the divine sexual act. Often the comfort level is such that it allows a complete physical and mental relaxation that will lead them to various states of awareness.

Asanas also promote exchanges of magnetic and vital energies, and facilitate the control of ejaculation. In this regard, Tantra disregards, at least at the beginning, the position most often used in the West, commonly known as the "missionary position" (*uttana bandka* in Sanskrit), in which the man lies on top of the woman. This position, according to the scholars, does not facilitate seminal control.

The Reason for the Positions

Let's try to understand the reason for the positions by means of an example. Start by inverting the missionary position and placing the woman on top. The advantage of this variation is that the woman (representing the goddess) can initiate the movements and control the experience. The man, on the other hand, although almost motionless, is better able to relax and let himself go.

This position also allows for an inverted union, in which the man adopts the position typically held by the woman, that is, lying on his back with his legs apart. The woman, in turn, performs the typical role of the man in the union and keeps her legs closed tight. This way the man can identify with female energy and reach a better understanding of his partner.

14

KAMA SUTRA: THE ART OF BEING GOOD LOVERS

Philosophy of the Kama Sutra

The Kama Sutra warns that although it does describe ways to achieve and provoke greater pleasure, it is harmony that keeps a couple together.

This harmony ensues when a man and a woman live as one single body and one single soul. This way their good deeds will be an example to all who know them, and therefore they will be happy both in this world and the hereafter.

The main reason for marital separation, and the chief cause of infidelity, is a lack of varied pleasures, which results in boredom and monotony in the sexual life of a couple.

The Sixty-Four

Sixty-Four *(Chatushshashti)* is the name of the part of the Sacred Scriptures dealing with the sexual union. Many say that its name is due to the fact that it has sixty-four parts, but others say that it has only eight parts subdivided into another eight. These parts are as follows:

1. The Caress
2. The Kiss
3. The Scratch
4. The Bite
5. The Sexual Union
6. The Erotic Screams
7. The Woman Who Assumes the Masculine Role
8. The Oral Union

Vatsyayana believed that this name was the result of coincidence and custom, since the Sixty-Four contains more than eight sections, such as the man's behavior during the love act and the various methods of sexual union.

Here is an example. The first subject addressed is the embrace. This bodily contact reflects the happiness of a man and a woman joined by love. According to the ancient scriptures, there are four types of embraces.

The most elementary type is the Embrace Through Touch. It takes place when a man feels the impulse of desire, and then seeks to touch a woman's body with his own.

When a woman bends over to pick up an object from the floor and her breasts lightly touch the body of her lover and he in turn caresses them with his hand, this is called the Embrace Through Penetration. These two types of embraces are used only by lovers who are not sure of their feelings or intentions toward each other.

If two lovers are walking through a shaded, pleasant garden, and their bodies rub against each other softly, this is called the Embrace Through Friction.

Lastly, when one lover presses passionately and forcefully against the body of the other, this is known as the Embrace Through Pressure. These last two forms are used only by those who have succumbed to the pleasure of Kama, and are willing to sail on together into the stormy ocean of desire.

The Rules of Life

The Rules of Life that were set by the Lord of Beings when he created man and woman are *Dharma, Artha,* and *Kama.*

The Dharma refers to the acquisition of religious merit. All laws having to do with religious life are part of the Dharma.

The Artha is related to material acquisitions, such as properties, real estate, jewels, and money. Whether someone amasses great riches or ends up living in poverty depends on how this discipline is observed.

Lastly is the Kama, which refers to everything having to do with love, desire, pleasure, and sexuality. The Kama Sutra is a collection of love proverbs. In India, every man must read the Kama Sutra before getting married.

The study of these three Rules of Life leads human beings to attain fulfillment and harmony and thereby to achieve happiness. They must be followed in order for one to learn to be whole. If one of the three rules is missing, the process is incomplete.

For this reason, the Kama Sutra is not only sex, as the West tends to see it, but it also includes forms and laws for appropriate behavior that both men and women ought to know, not only for the purpose of being experts on the Kama, but because knowledge of these arts will allow them to overcome any situation, anywhere and under any circumstances.

2

THE REALIZATION OF LOVE

15

THE ART
OF SACRED SEXUALITY
AND ITS PRACTICE

The Union

Within yoga's broad landscape, Tantra yoga is one of the most ancient disciplines. Many sustain that Tantra is found in the origin of all yoga, but there is no agreement in this regard. What is true is that the origins of these ancient Indian traditions are lost in the mist of history.

The word *yoga* comes from the Sanskrit root word *yug,* meaning "union." Yoga deals with the unions within human evolution up to the complete fusion with the Cosmic Entity or Divinity. This "union" is like mixing water with sugar—separately each has its own characteristics, taste, color, and appearance, but when mixed together they lose their differences, and we get sweet water—the water has been sugared, and the sugar is now a liquid. Yoga means the ultimate unification of the microcosm and macrocosm.

Tantra is the practical method for divine light to become manifest within each human heart in this material world. Tantra does not separate material life from spiritual life. A human being without his or her divine spark is not a complete human being, and that's where the most beautiful secret of all lies.

Tantra Yoga Exercises for a Wondrous Sexual Union

Tantra yoga sees sexual union as a union of body and soul, of male and female principles, of sexuality and spirituality. In Tantra, the most important sexual organ is the mind.

In order to enjoy a full sexual life, we need to pay attention to both the psychological aspects, since the mind plays a preponderant role in human relations, and the physical aspects, such as breathing exercises, yoga, proper nutrition, and a good attitude.

The more people understand this, the more they will stop consuming stimulants. The practice of yoga, or any of the various Taoist gymnastic exercises, is a powerful activator, free of costs and side effects, and accepted by modern sexology, which relies on and trusts the ancient exercises developed by Tantra and Taoism.

Ancient Practices

Here we will explain in detail some practices that will greatly help in achieving sexual fulfillment.

Primary Breathing

First, get "on all fours," with your hands and knees on the floor. Upon inhaling, lift your head, arch your back downward, and put out your belly. Upon exhaling, arch your back upward, lower your head, and sink in your belly. You may draw your pelvis close to the floor. Breathing should be slow and natural, not forced, to the rhythm of the expansion and contraction of the abdomen.

Then, while focusing, lie on your back and rest. You may place one hand on the area of your stomach to better observe the motions of the diaphragm.

Genital Breathing

Lying on your back, flex your legs and place your feet firmly on the floor. Then begin the genital breathing. This breathing consists of slow and deep abdominal respirations in which the belly is propelled forward during inhalation and drawn back in during exhalation.

Squat Breathing

Squat down with your heels firmly on the floor and the palms of your hands or the tips of your fingers braced on the floor. The arms are placed on the inside of the legs. Focus on the rhythmic motion of abdominal breathing.

During inhalation we bring the belly forward and bring it back in when exhaling. At each exhalation open your legs, imagining you are expelling air through the genitals. Then close your legs softly for another inhalation.

Breathing with Pelvic Motion

Lying on your belly, with your arms stretched forward, knees on the floor, and your toes braced securely on the floor, breathe deeply and slowly with your abdomen, enjoying the sensation and pushing your pelvis forward.

You don't need to perform the same exercises every day.

Classic Tantra Yoga Exercises

Here are some more practices that will greatly help in achieving sexual fulfillment.

The Flower

This exercise helps tighten the perineum or pelvic zone, which starts in the anus and ends in the genitalia. It is excellent for toning the anal sphincter, thus preventing hemorrhoids and other inconveniences by activating circulation, while also stimulating the urogenital system. In women it strengthens the walls of the vagina, thus preventing the possibility of anorgasmy. In men it decreases the likelihood of early ejaculation and impotence.

The man should sit on the floor with his back upright and his hands resting on his knees, with his palms facing up. He should first concentrate on his anal region by exerting pressure on his glutei. He should start with inhalations that are not too deep and hold the air in his chest while contracting his anus as tightly as possible. He should then extend the anal contraction forward until he feels a soft pull in his testicles inside the scrotum. Upon releasing the air, he should release the contraction and relax.

The woman should do likewise, but should extend the pressure exerted on her anus forward until she feels a slight pull on the labia of the vagina.

The Star

This exercise increases the sensitivity of the clitoris (the star) in women and the potency of the erection in men.

Drink several glasses of water on an empty stomach. Urinate after one hour, stopping and releasing the flow of urine at least ten times until the bladder is empty.

Then sit in the position described in the previous section, but this time concentrating on the urethral foramen (the hole where the urethra ends). After an average inhalation, contract the urethral foramen just as you would when you try to stop the flow of urine. Then relax the contraction and expel the air slowly.

In both exercises, contractions should be repeated as often as possible with the same retention of air. This will increase blood pressure in the area, which will cause a mild sexual excitement.

16

THE PLEASURE
OF A GOOD RELATIONSHIP

How to Achieve a Good
Sexual Relationship

For Taoists, the factor that truly unites a couple is a fully developed sexual relationship. That is why it is so important to achieve a deep mental and spiritual connection, both with one's mate and with one's own inner self.

Steps to Achieve Pleasure

Start by stimulating the erogenous zones. The first caresses should start at the arms and legs. It is advisable not to start at the genital area, because oftentimes this causes a certain sexual inhibition and the opportunity is lost to tap the energy of more stimulating spots.

The couple should start by massaging each other on the hands, wrists, feet, and ankles. Then move up to the arms and shoulders until reaching the chest. Continue up the legs and thighs until reaching the belly.

If this is done by the man, it is important that afterward the woman do it the same way, because these routes represent the main energy meridians.

Massages can be very exciting, especially if performed with some kind of moisturizing oil or cream. Lovers should concentrate on a pink light while they massage each other. The elements that allow us to surprise ourselves and surprise our lover are what differentiate a magical couple from your regular, garden-variety sexual relationship.

According to acupuncture, the zone that causes a better flow and lubrication in women is located about three inches above the ankle. This spot stimulates the awakening of the goddess.

The sensorial stimuli are accompanied by the visualization of the heart and a total focus on physical pleasure.

Little by little and without any kind of pressure, an impulse will emerge to very softly shift the caressing to the sexual organs.

For the woman, it will be very important to have certain areas stimulated continuously, such as the clitoris and the G-spot.

Disciplined concentration by the man will enable him to delay ejaculation and therefore maintain an erection for a longer time.

17

EROTIC INTELLIGENCE

Eroticism Is Intelligent

When a person touches another person's body, the brain receives stimuli at more than half a million receptors, which decode the information about the caressed object. During sexual relations, our body is stimulated all over. How can we take advantage of this erotic information within our reach?

Developing Erotic Intelligence

During sexual contact, concentration helps us recognize the body's various textures, which are infinite and subtle. There will be unexplored spaces—smooth, rough, flexible, wet, hot, cold, firm, delicate, thin, and thick spaces. It is important to activate all the senses in order to enjoy sex creatively.

Blind Touching

To stimulate the sense of touch, the partners, before making love, may perform the following exercise.

Take a handkerchief and cover your eyes, focusing all your attention on caressing each other. Investigating each other blindly sharpens our sense of hearing and helps us hear exciting whispers.

Savoring the Taste

There are around 10,000 taste buds that are used to differentiate the different flavors. How do they work? Inside the mouth, the taste buds are organized as follows: Sour flavors are registered on the sides of the tongue, bitter flavors on the back, salty flavors on the surface, and sweet flavors at the tip. The body issues different flavors in the course of a kiss. Recognizing each sensation generates greater satisfaction and ecstasy during the sexual act.

Changing Positions

Changing from one position to another during the sex act is very stimulating, but if lovers do not do it with sufficient erotic intelligence, it becomes merely a form of sexual athletics.

Smell and Touch

Place in water the petals of a flower, such as a jasmine or a rose, and wait until they dissolve on your fingers to create an instant sensual perfume. You can bring your partner to a state of rapture by touching him or her repeatedly with your perfumed hands.

Taste, Hearing, Touch, and Sight

While the partners stop for an instant to change positions, they can eat some foods that are arousing. They can eat these foods, observe them, and taste them while listening to the sounds inside the mouth. In addition, if these foods are placed on the body, they induce a strange and stimulating sensation. Foodstuffs may be varied: honey, cream, chocolate, sparkling wine—what is important is to allow ourselves to be playful.

By using erotic intelligence and creativity in each sexual act, you can take advantage of the whole capacity of your brain and truly become a genius in the art of making love.

18

THE SEXUAL TAO
AND MULTIPLE ORGASMS

Multiple Orgasms: Delight Multiplied

It is possible to expand the limits of pleasure and achieve more than one orgasm during each sexual encounter. Here we reveal the secrets of male and female multiple orgasms.

Sexual excitement may be induced in several ways: involuntarily, as the result of sexual fantasies or images, or by direct stimulation through physical contact.

The first sign that a person is getting excited is a rapid concentration of blood on the surface of the body, which accumulates in the erogenous zones—the penis, the clitoris, and the vagina. This causes an erection of the penis in men and vaginal lubrication in women.

To attain total pleasure, the partners must initiate the sexual relation consciously. When the man receives a sexual stimulus, his body releases a substance that causes the relaxation and subsequent erection of his penis. He must learn to maintain a state of relaxation in order to avoid reaching the point of ejaculation. The woman develops a better quality orgasm when the man succeeds in maintaining the erection for a longer time.

The Straight Path to Multiple Orgasms

In order to multiply satisfaction, the first step is to concentrate on the whole body and relax in order to generate a perfect chemistry. With practice, both lovers will be able to feel how each part of their bodies has a different sensitivity.

When the skin is stimulated by caresses, massages, or kisses, the body vibrates as a whole, like a single erogenous space—this is the principle that is going to enrich the erotic experience. It is important to know that with proper technique and the necessary knowledge of the body, men and women can achieve multiorgasmic experiences.

Different Forms of Pleasure

The mechanism of the orgasm can be explained as an explosive release of sexual energy. This explosion causes a muscular contraction throughout the body and subsequently results in complete relaxation.

The Single Orgasm

The single orgasm consists of a physiological sexual discharge that causes pleasure at that exact moment. In both sexes it can be induced through masturbation techniques, without the need for a partner. It lasts between two and ten seconds.

Multiple Orgasms

This state of pleasure is generated in a relationship where the partners perform the appropriate stimulation of their bodies. The experience of each bodily contraction is multiplied, with two to ten minutes of rest for men. In women the orgasms can be more continuous, with different intensity and regularity.

Orgasmic Chain Reaction

This is a sequence of continuous orgasms to the point where they become one single long orgasm, consisting of six to twelve orgasms nonstop. In this case, the man ejaculates only during the last period of orgasmic contractions. In the woman, once she starts, the release of pleasure won't stop. When the woman controls the orgasmic chain reaction, the moment in which the erotic session ends depends on her wishes. Orgasmic control will depend on psychological and emotional aspects, provided the woman has been able to achieve this maximum stage of utmost pleasure.

Refractory Period

This is the resting period that ensues after an orgasm—it is the time needed by the body to recover after the orgasmic discharge and to be able to become excited again. In the case of women, this phase can last between one and ten minutes, depending on the lover's suitable stimulation. In men, the refractory stage lasts longer, between fourteen to twenty minutes, depending on the appropriate motivation by their mates. The refractory period will also depend on the age of the lovers, how much they have practiced, and the experiences they have had together.

Sexual pleasure is unlimited when the mind is liberated through the true knowledge of all our sexual potential.

19

POSITIONS OF
THE KAMA SUTRA

Sexual Yoga

The positions of the Kama Sutra excite imagination and enhance pleasure. We will explain the positions in the following pages.

Unlike Chinese bedroom books, which emphasize methods, the Kama Sutra is devoted to classifying sexual relations with astonishing attention to detail and postures, but leaving ample room for spontaneity, which belongs in the spiritual realm.

The Wheelbarrow

The partners get ready to make love at the edge of the bed. The woman props her forearms on the bed while the man "lifts" her by the legs and places himself standing up behind her to penetrate her while holding her thighs.

Stimulation and pleasure are concentrated in the partners' genitals, but it is the man who sets the rhythm of the act, drawing her body toward his.

Her legs may close up or open up wide, as preferred by the partners, who may engage in changing the angle. The variety of motions (circular, ascending and descending) allowed by this posture is astonishing and very exciting. The sensations are intense.

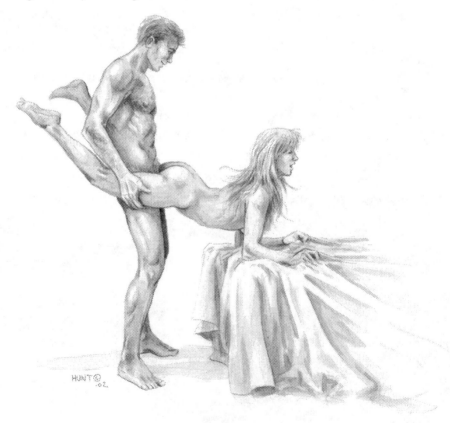

The Hammock

To perform the sexual act in this position, it is advisable for the man to sit on a hard surface (not a bed) with his legs flexed and grabbing the back side of his knees. The woman, with her legs open, allows herself to be penetrated by accommodating herself in the space remaining between his legs and his trunk, with the man's arms surrounding her legs.

The man presses his knees against the body of his mate, drawing her to himself and causing their bodies to engage in a rhythmic motion while kissing her breasts, which are close to his face. The pleasure of breast stimulation is delightful for the woman and arousing for the man. The woman, with her neck bent backward in a gesture of submission, enjoys the incredible pleasure provided by her mate.

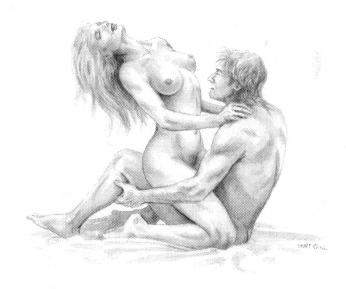

The Mold

With her legs together and tucked in, the woman lies on her side and relaxes her head backward while the man penetrates her, whether through the vagina or the anus. This is an excellent position for anal sex. The woman who dares to live this anal sex experience will be able to complete and integrate her body as a perfect universe to love and enjoy without stopping to check on the quality or quantity of eroticism.

The moves must be soft and coordinated and penetration deep and slow. Both bodies fit each other perfectly, as would two pieces of a jigsaw puzzle. The fact that the woman's legs are held together combined with squeezing can exert an ideal pressure on the penis and at the same time cause a pleasant friction on the clitoris.

This last aspect makes it an ideal position for women who have problems reaching orgasm. They only have to relax and enjoy it fully.

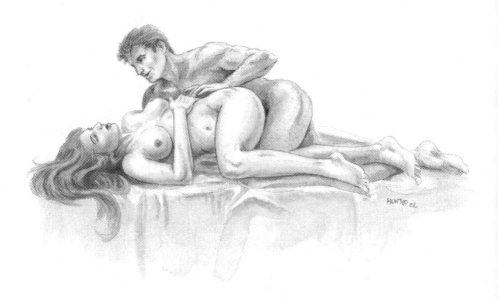

The Trapeze

The man sits with his legs open and his partner, on top of him, opens up to a slow penetration, feeling fulfilled and giving herself up to her lover to be complemented.

The man takes the woman by the wrists while he feels an overwhelming joy toward her. Then he leans back, relaxing slowly until he falls back completely. It is important for the woman to remain relaxed and to give herself up to the strength of her lover, who draws her in with his arms and engages in the powerful thrusts needed for the act of lovemaking.

This position combines several movements. It requires agility and a relaxed surrender on the part of the woman, and strength and skill on the part of the man. Both balance and complement each other.

This position is ideal for changing the routine and for experiencing new emotions.

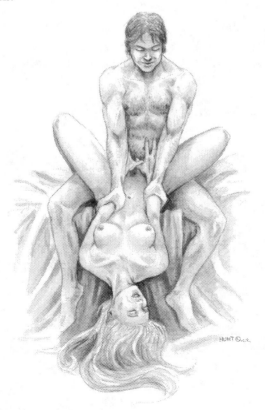

The Mirror of Pleasure

The woman lies on her back and lifts her legs in a vertical position while her breathing betrays the joy of showing her wet and longing parts to her partner. She then lets him hold her legs, with her partner kneeling at the end of her body and propping his other arm on the floor. The man penetrates her, subdues her, and controls her, varying the direction of the penetration and the opening of the legs.

Their faces can't get near each other and the man's hands can do very little in this position, which generates an extremely arousing anxiety. The two bodies run the race together to reach orgasm, bestowing on each other the most varied gestures of pleasure, sensuality, affection, and eroticism.

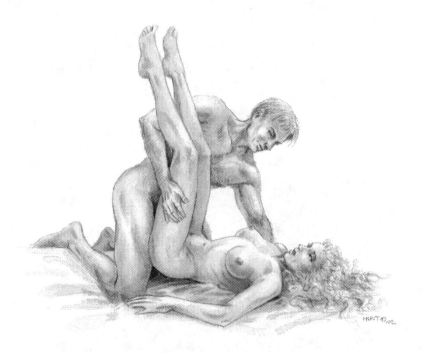

The Dragonfly

To perform the sexual act in this position, the partners must lie on their sides on a flexible and comfortable place, such as a bed or a sofa. The woman lies on her side with her back turned to her partner, and he mounts her from the back. This way, the bodies fit each other in a position that is ideal for very affectionate couples who enjoy demonstrating the tenderness they feel toward each other.

With a bit of skill combined with much excitement, the woman takes her flexed outer leg and places it on the man's coccyx, thus opening the door to pleasure. The man penetrates her by using his lover's leg as an erotic lever bracing on the support of his hip.

The flattering words the man is able to whisper in his partner's ear, because it is so close to his mouth, provide the perfect compliment to achieve the utmost delight, in addition to ardent kisses. The woman, upon just listening to him, lets herself be taken over by the rhythm of his kisses, while she shows her lover all the effects his potency has on her through her expressions of intense pleasure.

Penetration goes halfway, which is why the pleasure is enhanced by the desire to make penetration deep and cause the explosion of the most exciting orgasm.

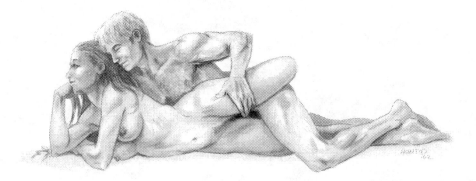

The Screw

Nothing is more advisable to a woman who finds it difficult to reach orgasm than assuming positions that press on the clitoris while the vagina is penetrated. Orgasm always comes in this position, and multiple experiences of pleasure become concrete and unforgettable feelings for the woman.

She lies down by the edge of the bed and places her flexed legs to one side of her body (each woman will know which side is most comfortable for her). This enables her to keep the clitoris trapped between the best allies she has to reach the prized orgasm—the labia of her vagina.

The woman can contract and relax that entire region, while the man, kneeling in front of her, penetrates her softly. To turn this position into a true delicacy, it is suitable for the man, while penetrating her, to caress her breasts and for the woman to groan with pleasure to arouse her partner.

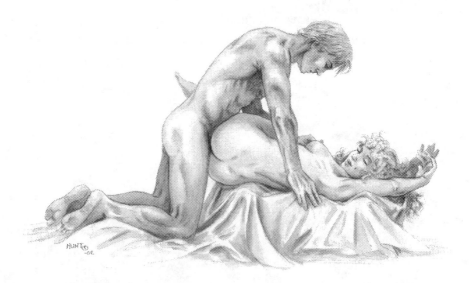

The Amazon

This position puts the woman in a totally active position. She places herself on top of the man and sets the rhythm of the sexual relation by bracing her feet on the floor. It is ideal for active women who are a bit domineering and like to set the sexual rhythm in a relationship.

For the man, this is an extraordinary experience because in this position he can incorporate the yin energy, which is more passive, and in addition be able to relax in the course of the sexual act. In turn he can touch her breasts and pull the hair of his mate while she moves.

The visual angle made possible by this variation is one of the most exciting angles for the man, since he is able to see close at hand each thrust he performs on his partner. And the woman will get much pleasure from the idea of knowing that she is in control of the sexual act and that the man knows it.

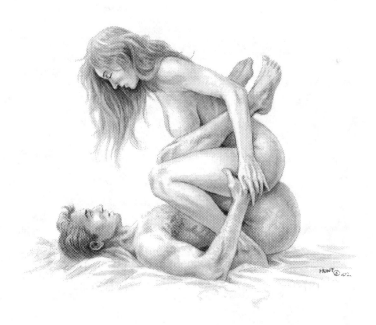

The Easy Chair

Leaning on a big, comfortable cushion or pillow, the man sits with his legs flexed and a bit open. The woman sits comfortably on the space he's formed with his body. In this position, the protective feelings of both partners come to the fore.

Assisted by his arms and hands, the man finds the satisfactory point of encounter for both and places his partner on his erection, controlling the sexual rhythm.

Her legs are braced on the shoulders of her mate, who has his head trapped and wrapped between her thighs. The man can touch her clitoris while he forcefully grabs her by her waist.

The distance between the faces and the daring aspect of this proposal endow this position with an extremely sensual quality.

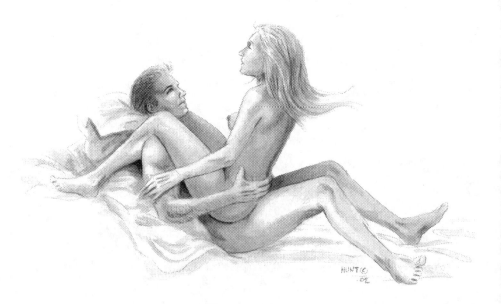

The Sleepy Woman

The woman lies on her side and the man mounts her from the back in order to penetrate her. She stretches a leg backward and wraps it around his waist. This position is ideal for well-endowed men who always had experiences in the traditional position, and for very flexible women who want to place their whole body at the disposal of their mate.

Additionally, it fulfills several longings of fantasy-driven minds. First of all, she is in front of him and at the same time has access to his face and neck, and he has access to her face and neck. Secondly, he has comfortable access to her clitoris and is able to touch and feel the breasts of his lover.

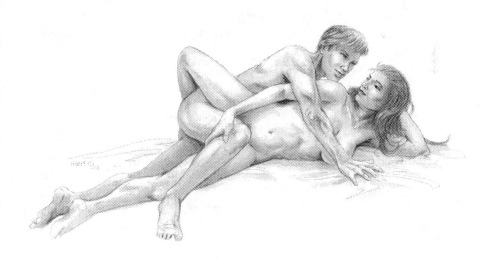

The Surprise

In this position the man must be standing up to grab the woman from behind, penetrate her, and at the same time take her by the hips in a sensual manner and with a certain degree of domination. She relaxes her whole body and places her hands on the floor in an attitude of surrender and of confidence in her partner. The man "surprises" the woman from behind, setting the erotic rhythm almost completely.

For her, pleasure is concentrated because of the opening angle of the vagina, which, being narrow, provokes a very intense, pleasant sensation. For him, the most powerful sensation expands upward from the glans, which comes into and out of the vagina at will and caresses the clitoris in the most daring moves as it comes out. In addition, the man's visual field covers her anus, her buttocks, and her back, zones that are very erogenous for many people. The domination exerted by the man on the woman together with her complete relaxation may foster playfulness in the man, who while seducing his lover is able to play around with her anus. If she already knows the experience, the woman may approach the sensation of pleasure caused by her lover's anal penetration.

This position is ideal for those who love the most savage and primitive forms of sexual intercourse.

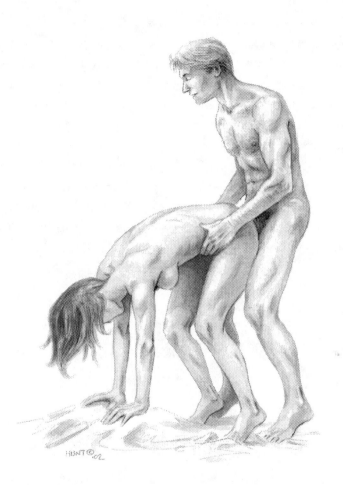

The Medusa

The partners should kneel on a comfortable surface, though not as soft as a bed. In this position, the man surrenders to the woman's will. She descends on his penis and introduces it into her vagina whenever she wishes. Before penetration, they may kiss, rub each other's breasts, hug, caress each other's back, and place the glans in her vagina and rub it against the clitoris, creating a pleasant and very different sensation, an almost unique one. After being very much desired, the penetration will come with infinite pleasure at the end.

In the course of the love act, if he can't surrender patiently to her moves, he'll be able to set the rhythm by grabbing her by the waist and drawing her body to his.

Since the partners are face to face, this offers the exciting opportunity to observe each other, rejoice together, talk, and kiss each other on the mouth until achieving the much desired orgasm.

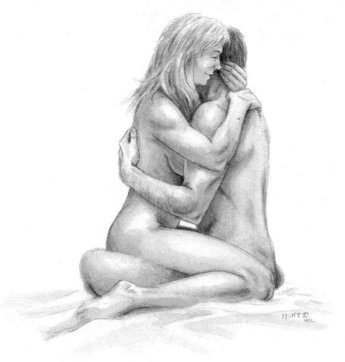

The Fusion

In this position, the man sits down, tilting his body slightly backward, supporting it by bracing his hands on the bed on each side of his body. The legs may be stretched or bent, depending on the partners' comfort. The heads of both partners should be relaxed. The woman assumes the active role on this occasion, passing her legs over her lover and supporting herself by bracing her arms behind her body.

To be totally successful in this position, stimulation must be intense, since during penetration this position prevents manual contact and contact of the mouths of the partners.

The woman sets the rhythm and establishes the genital encounter with a very marked motion. It is essential to have the clitoris take full advantage of the impacts with her lover's body in order to maintain the excitement until the moment she decides to explode with pleasure, provided her lover keeps the rhythm with a good erection.

The look is a fundamental component, but so is sensual and provocative communication, since erotic words provide a very strong sexual charge to the love act. Both resources (looks and words) can be unbelievable weapons used to enjoy this position and achieve a complete "fusion."

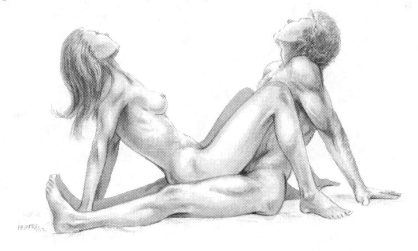

Possession

As its name indicates, this position is captivating and has a certain degree of suggestion, especially for the woman. The man can use all his sexual magnetism and enjoy his own energy in this posture.

The woman lies on her back with her legs open, waiting for her partner to penetrate her, while he sits down and holds her by her shoulders to regulate the motion. Their legs become intertwined in a sensual and pleasant manner.

The male organ penetrates and withdraws, deviating its movement downward, since the body of the woman is slightly higher than the body of the man. He can then explore the woman's G-spot and all of her genital area in order to give his partner everything she loves.

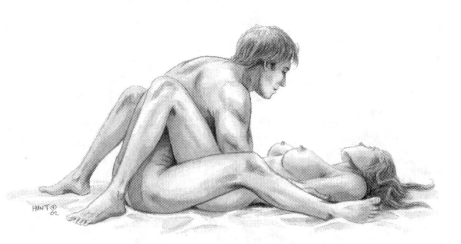

Face to Face

This is the most classic and universal position known in the art of making love. It provides a lot of security for couples in which the woman needs the man's bodily, sexual, and emotional protection.

The state of being face to face makes for a large number of variations to this position, which makes it an attractive and exciting one. The mobility of the hands, the closeness of the faces, and the comfort of the bodies are some of the advantages that made it famous.

The lovers should not fear trying new types of contact during the love act in this position. She can touch her mate's glutei and anal areas. He can rub her clitoris or allow her to do it herself. The legs of both partners may be closer together in order to create a certain degree of difficulty in the penetration.

This is a position that many lovers identify with the love and romance they experienced at the beginning of their life as a couple. It is worth it to experience it at the various stages of their sexual life and to profit to the utmost from all its advantages.

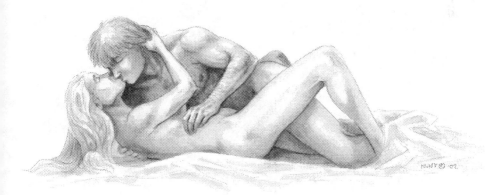

Face-to-Face Variation

This is the same classic position, but the difference, perhaps more exciting, is that the woman assumes the active and dominating role. This
variation of the "face to face" is a position that favors women who can't
reach orgasm easily because they need a very active and direct stimulation of the clitoris and labia.

In this variation of the love act, the woman can rub her clitoris
against the body of her lover, and, due to her dominating position, can
move easily and with greater bodily freedom. Additionally, the man can
touch with joy his mate's buttocks and play around with his fingers in
search of the complete satisfaction of both partners.

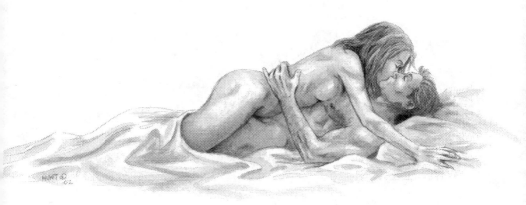

Taming the Horse

While sitting comfortably, the man receives his mate, who fits into his body by sitting on his erection.

In this position, the woman can seduce her lover in many ways. One of them is to touch and expertly caress his genital area. When the male organ reaches its maximum erection, she takes it and assists in the penetration. Then, with her hands, she sensually cooperates in the sexual maneuvers.

If both lovers desire, the man can impose his will by pressing the woman slowly against his member while looking her in the eyes.

The passion of the embrace, the playful games with the tongue, the kisses, and the soft massages or caresses on each other's backs cause shudders in the partner and are some of the additions that make this position a very sensual one.

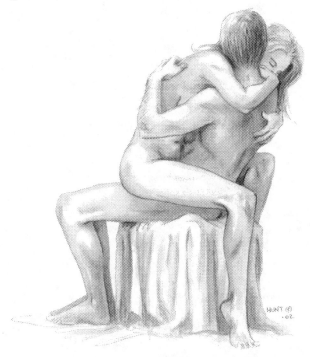

The Subjected Man

In spite of the name, this is one of the Kama Sutra positions that is most preferred by male lovers. Male submission can be totally sexually stimulating for a couple, especially for those partners who have been in a relationship for a long time.

The man lies down, surrendering his body to his partner's will. The encounter may start with caresses and kisses performed by her on him. He always remains in the same position, but she may eventually turn her back to him. The woman controls the movements by aiding herself with her arms. Deep penetration is made possible by this position.

It is very erotic for the couple to have their eyes meet when she shows her face over her shoulder. In addition, the man has easy access to his lover's anal area and buttocks. It is the woman who regulates the speed of the sexual rhythm and of their movements. As she moves, both can enjoy the anal and genital stimulation of this position, which is a very adequate variation of the love act.

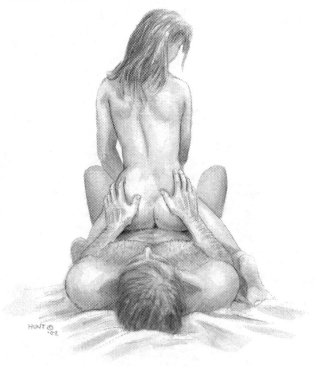

The Delight

This position should be performed in a comfortable and very intimate place, one that allows for playfulness in freedom. The woman should get close to the edge of a bed or chair. Her lover kneels down in order to penetrate his mate with his genital area at the same height as her vagina.

The woman, feeling very relaxed, throws her body backward and opens her legs to receive her lover. At the same time, she surrounds his body with her legs. She can set the sexual rhythm in this position, but if both have a motion that is harmonic, full, and open, the mutual delight will be explosive.

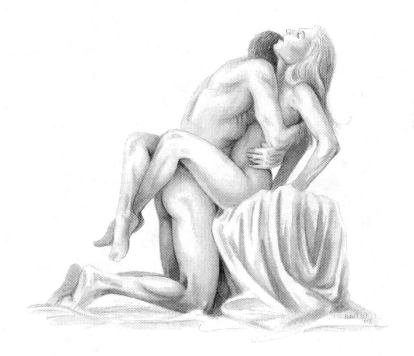

The Deep One

The advantage of this position is that is makes total penetration possible, hence its name. The woman, with her legs raised and open, waits
for her lover to penetrate her. Then she raises her legs to the utmost
until they reach above his shoulders. The man then braces his hands on
the floor to regulate the rhythm of the act.

Many women may feel this position is complicated, uncomfortable,
or painful, but it has to be experienced. The excitement felt by the man
in this position is moving, and the pleasure that can be shared is extraordinary.

This position provides an absolute penetration and a unique genital
contact when the testicles are placed on the glutei and the clitoris is
pressed by the opening of the legs.

The difficulty in kissing and the distance between the faces may be
interesting for the partners when they draw near each other's mouths
and feel limited by their bodies. Both can play around with the irony of
flexibility and the love they feel in the need to get near, while having to
contain each other.

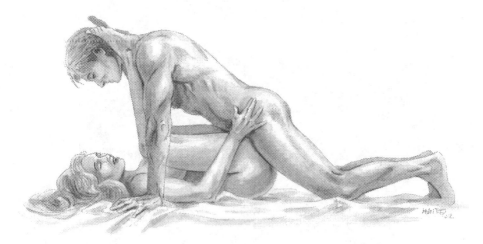

The Windmill's Blade

In this position, the woman lies on her back with her legs open to be penetrated by her lover. He penetrates her facing her legs. The difference in sensation is remarkable: the clitoris and the labia are in full contact with the male pelvis and genital area. The most intense penetration is achieved through deep circular motions.

The fact that the lovers can't see each other's faces gives a mysterious flavor to this position. The novelty of the caresses surprises and enriches the relationship. The woman can caress her mate's buttocks or softly stick her nails on the back side of his knees. The man can attempt to suck the feet of his lover and lightly bite her toes. They can both also draw their hands near the genitals that are fusing passionately with each other.

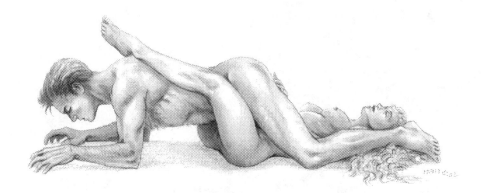

The Acrobatic Position

This position is recommended for couples training in the art of love-making who have flexible bodies and are willing to live very intense experiences full of marvelous motions.

The man lies down, relaxed but excited, with his penis totally erect. The woman sits facing away from him and lets him penetrate her while flexing her knees and tilting her body backward so her lover can perform deep penetrations of her vagina.

To activate the motions needed for the act, the woman should lift her waist and relax on her mate. The man thus has easier access to her clitoris and genital area.

She should relax the rest of her body. The decline in muscle tone for each area of the body is what makes this position so special, since the woman can reach an explosive orgasm that will leave her exhausted.

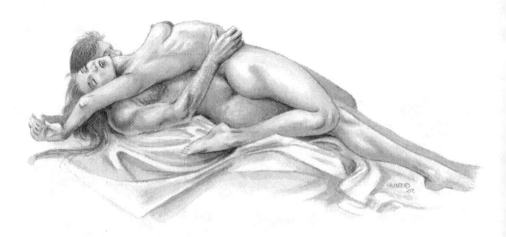

The Bow

This position is a variation of the "face to face," but it modifies sensations to the extreme. The woman is lying on her back with her legs open and flexed, bracing her arms behind her shoulders. When her partner is ready to penetrate her, she raises her hips and perches herself on the flexed legs of her mate.

The pleasure she receives is focused on the deep penetration and especially on feeling her whole vaginal and abdominal areas covered and protected by the heat of her lover's skin.

When this position stays firm, lovers experience formidable pleasure during orgasm, especially if, by keeping adequate sexual rhythm, they achieve a synchronized climax.

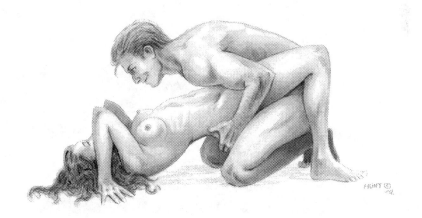

Savage Furor

The name of this position is due to the fact that it allows the man to develop and fantasize with all of his instinctive potential, while his lover surrenders to him almost completely in the love act.

For this position, the woman kneels with her flexed hands and her bent knees on the floor. The man places himself behind her, in the same position but covering his lover's body.

In order to be more comfortable, the woman can support her body by placing her arms on the floor, bending her waist, and opening her legs to expose her vulva. It is very useful for both to put a big cushion or pillow beneath their knees to protect them.

The man takes the woman by the waist and penetrates her deeply through the vagina or the anus, according to the couple's needs and desires. He can add to the penetration by touching the breasts of his mate. Or, if he wishes to achieve a special kind of satisfaction, he can perform the penetration more slowly and brace an arm on the floor in order to sustain the fused bodies in the air.

The almost complete control exerted by the man adds a very exciting component to this position.

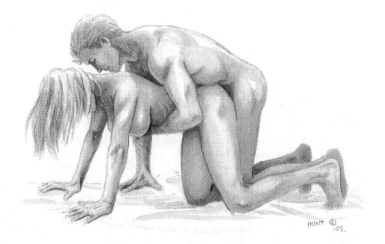

The Catapult

This position is a valuable source of pleasure, since it puts the man's body in contact with areas of the woman's body that usually remain untouched in more traditional positions.

The man kneels and receives his partner while she places her glutei over the legs of her lover. The woman can stretch her legs over the man's torso or bend her knees by placing the soles of her feet on his chest. This is very exciting for the man when the woman is able to play on his chest with the soles of her feet.

The man has easy access to his lover's clitoris, which is why he is able to stimulate her genital area with his hands. In turn, the woman can perform a sensual motion with the shifting and raising of her hips. The rhythm is set by both partners, depending on the desire, passion, and flexibility of each.

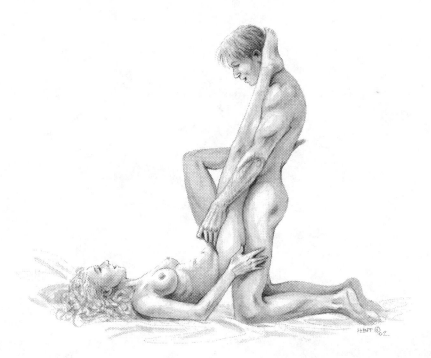

The Total Embrace

This position promotes passionate and creative sex, in which bodily contact is complete. To have sex in this position, both lovers must feel a sense of great surrender.

Both are naked, standing up and face to face to love each other. She goes up her partner's body and hangs by his shoulders in order to embrace her lover's body with her arms and legs. He grabs her by the buttocks and draws her toward his body in order to penetrate her.

The rhythm of the love act can be set in two ways: up and down or back and forward, depending on the intensity, surrender, time, potency, and the need to experience a vigorous erotic rhythm.

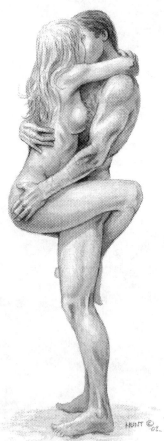

Variation of the Subjected Man

In this variation of the "subjected man" position, the woman stretches her body backward, bracing her arms on the arms of her partner and stretching her legs forward. This way the man can easily stimulate the breasts of his lover, and the woman can place her buttocks on her partner in order to perform deep circular motions.

In this position, penetration is not complete, but it is a very powerful game prior to a more intense act of lovemaking. If she keeps up her sensual motions, the woman will oftentimes attain a more explosive orgasm.

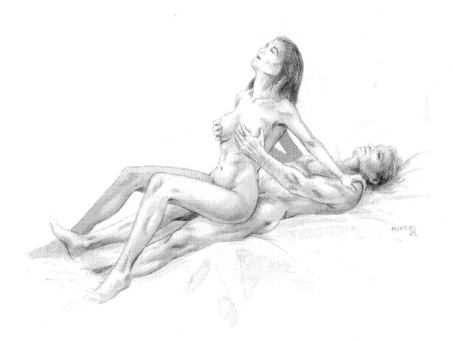

Variation of the Fusion

Here, the rhythm of the sexual act is set by the woman through the motion that she can best regulate and perform in this position: the up-and-down oscillation.

If the man relaxes and supports his whole body while the woman gets up slightly, the fusion causes a deeper penetration.

Her hands can touch her lover's chest during the love act. The man can stimulate the clitoris, and the woman can increase the pleasure for both by performing deep tactual stimulation of his erogenous zone.

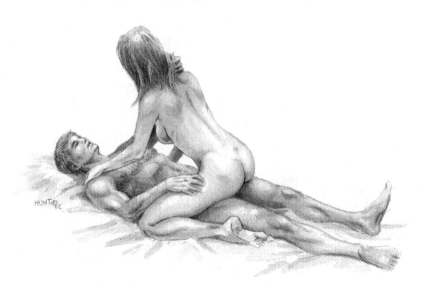

The Teaspoon

This is an excellent position for anal sex. With her legs together and tucked in, the woman can press against the man's penis and feel it more intensely while she lies on her side and relaxes her head backward.

Penetration can be anal or vaginal, as preferred by the couple. If movements are soft and coordinated, and penetration deep and slow, the bodies fit together and fuse as if they were pieces of a jigsaw puzzle.

This position reinforces the friction on the clitoris, which is satisfying for her and tremendously exciting for him.

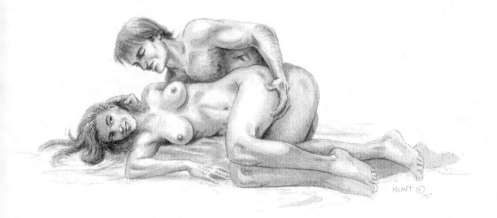

3

THE

EXPANSION

OF LOVE

20

DISCOVERING
EROTIC CHEMISTRY

How to Spark Sexual Chemistry

In a couple, there are several reasons why the chemistry of passion does not work the same as time goes by as it did at the beginning of the relationship. These include stress, financial problems, changes in schedule when a child is born, routine, and lack of communication.

But it also happens that two lovers, after a certain period, lose sexual desire without any apparent cause. Why does the sexual chemistry that prevailed at the beginning of the relationship cease to exist? How can intense eroticism be kept alive or elicited as time goes by?

Sexuality is an art and the highest point of pleasure is not the orgasm, but rather a state of ecstasy for an unlimited time. You need not be a sexual athlete to achieve this.

Elements That Fuel the Flame

Keeping the flame alive is not easy, but it can be learned as matter-of-factly as when one begins loving a person through mutual contact and knowledge.

Look for Complicity

Be alert to your mate's looks and thoughts. Find the proper moment, anywhere and at any time, to let that person know something with the wink of an eye. Use secret codes that have meaning for the two of you. Tempt your partner to make love in some "forbidden" place or one that will bring much excitement for you both.

Celebrate Different Events in Intimacy

Remember moments in which you both had that chemistry and honor those moments with a toast. Use flowers, special fragrances, and candles to create a romantic atmosphere and to increase excitement to the utmost.

Watch How You Make Love

Do you make love mechanically as if it were just one more routine, or do you surrender without limitations? Pay attention to your lover's reactions, looks, and gestures, and caress his or her whole body with a great discharge of eroticism with each move.

Do What Excites Your Partner

Find out whether you do everything that your mate really likes. If that's not the case, try to. It might just be that whispering erotic stories in his or her ear or dressing up in a certain special way opens the path to excitement.

Stimulate and Sexually Provoke Your Lover

Provoke your lover sexually, and then draw back and do something else until your partner seeks you out, burning with desire. Playfulness is an element that generates a lot of passion in one's partner.

Don't Forget to Communicate

When you are with your partner, express your love for him or her, and reveal the burning in your heart for him or her. This constant affirmation is an indispensable step in maintaining the chemistry of love.

21

TRAVELING THE LOVE MAPS

Pleasure Maps

When we remember our sexual experiences, the files from the past don't always provide us with exciting images. These "post cards" generate different emotions, sometimes even frustration or impotence. These negative memories provoke in us a deep fear of repeating a particularly unsatisfactory sexual experience.

Recent studies have discovered the "brain map" that organizes acquired knowledge. By means of these mental plans, we are able to consciously replace undesirable data pwith more pleasant information. We can indeed develop our erotic intelligence in order to feel pleasure again without associating our new sexual experiences with bad memories.

How Erotic Maps Are Charted

The workings of these brain organizers also allow us to chart our "sex maps"—new routes to pleasure, connected directly to the sense detectors we use in the sex act. The purpose is to modify negative information and chart new love maps. There are many ways to do this, but the simplest is by using visualization, logic, and emotional memory.

New Pleasure Routes

Men and women have different erotic zones. To find them and order them in accordance with the feelings they give evoke, we suggest performing the following exercise.

Select a photograph of your whole body. Make a copy (enlarge it if small) and paste it on a white sheet of paper.

Mark each place of your body that causes a positive or a negative sensation. Use different colors according to your personal criteria.

After marking these areas, write down the feelings they cause. The parts of the body may be marked with an arrow, as in a road map, writing down the stimulation felt in that particular zone. The most sensitive area in women is their breasts; to be more exact, their nipples, which are the first to react to sexual stimuli. Other major female erogenous zones are the mons veneris, the entrance to the vagina, the anal region, and the clitoris (the organ of pleasure par excellence). In men, the erogenous zones are located in the pelvis, but also in other areas such as the mouth and the neck. It is important to work these maps in a conscientious manner and see what changes have occurred in the performance of the sex act.

In the future you will be able to revise your erotic map to add new associations of sensations with bodily areas.

Visualizing and associating the erogenous zones with concrete feelings (and putting them into words) causes a conscious change in memory.

22

TECHNIQUES
FOR BEING TENDER

Love Food: Hugs and Kisses

There are different kinds of kisses, as many as the relationships in which they take place and the people who give them: kissing with a look, kissing at a distance, awakening kisses, magical kisses, spontaneous kisses, virtual kisses, passionate kisses, commitment kisses, faked kisses, ardent kisses . . . and so on.

The most common hugs are good-bye hugs, arrival hugs, re-encounter hugs, affectionate hugs, endless hugs, and friendly hugs. Which hugs and kisses would you like to give or receive? Who is the person you want to hug and kiss right now? Do you think you could have ever prevented a separation with a timely hug or kiss?

The purpose of hugs and kisses is to show deep affection, passion, fellowship, friendship, sexual needs, protection, mercy, consolation, wisdom, power, or love.

What do we feel when we kiss or hug? Excitement, appreciation, self-esteem, safety, approval, contentment, strength, devotion, spirituality, protection, enthusiasm, and happiness. Kissing is psychologically related to the most primitive contact in human beings and reminds us subconsciously of all our oral needs, such as the need for food, its enjoyment, flavor, what has been wished for, and what has been rejected—everything related to survival.

Practice the art of kissing every day. Prepare a list of all the people whom you would like to hug or kiss, and the reason for it. Then try to understand why you don't do it on a daily basis in each case.

If one of the first people on your list is your partner, awaken that person with a kiss. If your mate does not live with you, make a phone call and greet him or her with a kiss, send a message with kisses every day, talk at least one minute a day, or do it by e-mail including the words *kiss* and *hug*.

Try to do the same thing every day with all the people on your list. Choose the most appropriate kiss or hug depending on the relationship and degree of closeness.

Love Ritual

When you feel depressed, when you're having problems with your partner, when you have low self-esteem and don't feel loved or desired, remind yourself that this is all a reflection of your thoughts and feelings of love for your own self. Then perform the following exercise.

Choose a quiet place and relax. You may fill the room with the pleasant scent of incense or perfume. Listen to quiet music and try to dress as comfortably as possible.

Lie down wherever you feel most at ease. Visualize each cell of your skin and imagine that they turn into small kisses with different characteristics and colors, for example red kisses, sweet kisses, healthy kisses, loving kisses, ardent kisses, and sensual kisses. Imagine that you hug your own body and that you caress yourself, or place your arms around yourself. When you finally feel that you really love yourself, imagine the person you desire in front of you. Kiss and hug that person in your imagination.

You'll be able to see how the energy of your love can do miracles in your relationships. Now you only have to wait, because hugs and kisses will come to you.

23

THE LAW OF
LOVING ATTRACTION
AND HOW TO PRACTICE IT

Removing Sexual Blocks

All human beings at some time in their lives have wondered: Shall I be able to please this person who has so kindled my fancy? Shall I ever feel the pleasure that I so desire?

To answer this question in the affirmative, we must feel that throughout our sexual experiences we have developed enough self-confidence to control our own bodies and feelings with complete freedom.

But currently, we live in a fast-moving world that leads us to doubt our capacity to love. That is why it is important to know that there are erotic self-suggestion techniques, based on self-hypnosis, to release the mind and the body from the stress factors that cause a person to not be able to relate naturally to their own sexuality.

These techniques are very simple and may be performed in approximately fifteen minutes at any time of the day.

How to Practice Erotic Self-Suggestion

The first thing you have to do is try to evoke your sexual blocks and write them down in a notebook so you don't forget. It is not always easy to identify these conflicts consciously. In order to evoke them successfully, you should relax your body and remember the problem with all your senses and with a clear mind.

There are different self-suggestion methods to achieve complete relaxation. The quickest and most advisable one is to focus your eyes on a point until your eyelids relax and fall by their own weight. At that moment, your whole body is devoted to investigating whatever you are trying to know and solve.

After you achieve this state, it is important to repeat the following phrase to yourself mentally: "Each time I close my eyes, I'm going to relax and achieve an ever more pleasant state to be aware of all of my being." This way, the more you practice self-suggestion, the more easily you'll achieve an ever deeper state of visualization and self-knowledge.

Your memory will be complete if you check what you remember with each of your senses: taste, smell, sight, touch, and hearing. To call forth the taste you felt at the moment you were experiencing the block, you should ask yourself, for example, "Was the taste pleasant, bitter, sweet, or salty?" Then you should perform the same exercise with the smells: "What aroma did I perceive? Was it unpleasant, stale, musty, like plastic, or like a perfume?"

To the extent that you remember successfully with each sense, you will be able to dissociate it from the bad experience and eventually remove the block completely.

USE THE KNOWLEDGE OF THE TAO TO BECOME AN IRRESISTIBLE LOVER

The Tao of Sexual Magnetism

Your body is wrapped around me,
Your words fascinate me
like a love spell.
I'm so vulnerable
to your look that the farther I get from you,
the stronger the magnetism
of your presence inside me.

Who has not been subdued, at least once in their life, by the fascination cast by people who possess an indefinable charisma?

Every object has its own magnetic field. Human beings possess an especially active magnetic charge, and the erotic field stands out among the fields of action that magnetic energy can influence.

All human beings have the power to issue forth streams of the vital energy that gives us life itself, acknowledging that these waves can indeed influence the people we desire sexually, even at a distance. A person's magnetic field acts directly on another in a situation of trance or suggestion. But to make use of this powerful magnetic current and be able to transmit this attraction to others, you need to develop your own powers of suggestion.

Understanding Sexual Magnetism

A person can have three kinds of natural sexual magnetism:

1. A physiological action known as "animal magnetism."
2. An action of a more subtle nature that acts at a distance through will and thought.
3. An action produced by external factors: the resonance of one's voice, a special presence, suggestive behavior, a certain look, and other special gestures.

Suggestion and Self-Suggestion

Suggestion is a physiological process that, if you learn how to control it, can even cause another person to follow your orders, because each idea that is understood by the brain tends to become an action.

Is it possible to use suggestion in our conversations or contacts with other people? Yes, but in order to achieve this, it is indispensable to have blind confidence in ourselves. A person is as he or she thinks. That is why we must think intensely of the idea (and the sexual charge) that we wish to transmit to the other person.

Suggestion may also be defined as a self-affirmation intended to reinforce an idea with respect to oneself or to other people. By means of self-convincing, it is possible to give rise to thoughts loaded with strength, greatness, and power. If these powers are exercised, little by little the ideas of power and sensuality that we want to transmit to others become fixed in our own selves, stimulating the subconscious.

A Simple Suggestion Exercise

Every day, when you get up or go to bed, you should repeat to yourself the following affirmation: "I have confidence in myself and great magnetism in my dealings with others."

Here is another possible affirmation: "I am liberating myself of all my inner conflicts and I attract sexually whomever I desire."

It is important that you repeat these sentences for some time, with the absolute certainty that the magnetism you are developing will be irresistibly seductive for any mortal being.

25

TECHNIQUES FOR A PERFECT AND EFFECTIVE FIRST TIME

The Keys to an Intense Sexual First Time

Before the first erotic encounter, everybody feels a certain amount of fear. There are some people who communicate with each other through a certain affinity and attract each other physically at first sight, but how can they be sure that their first sexual encounter won't be a false spontaneous combustion that will end up totally extinguishing their passion?

If you have already experienced too many disappointments with partners who seemed to be sexual wild animals, and turned out to be a fiasco, here you'll find a short list of advice so that your next love encounter won't become a bad combination of hormones.

Advice for Women

1. Don't go by your first impression in the case of a man who is very passionate and, like a caged lion, wants to touch you as soon as you get near, especially if he tries to do it the first time you have a date with him. In general, you should consider a congenial man who is not too bold, because he is surely someone who will respect your needs.

2. Go with your instincts. Consider your own desire to hug him or protect him. If this impulse arises spontaneously, don't repress it.

3. Some men handle excitement very well and know how to seduce effectively, but others don't. The best thing is not to let yourself feel frustrated after an erotic encounter, because a failed first experience can prevent a full future relationship.

4. Before the first erotic encounter, see if he pays attention to you. A receptive man will listen attentively and look at your body discreetly but with desire. He may not take the initiative, but will observe your hand gestures and the way you look at him, and his movements will be calm and self-assured.

5. Another thing to take into account is that many men expect you to make the first physical move. For example, this type of man will wait until you give him a signal that he is well received, or for you to sit closer to him in the car, or move your body forward while you share dinner, sitting face to face in a restaurant.

6. If you really desire his body, try kissing him. If he's the right man, his caresses will be soft and sensual and won't go directly to your breasts or other erogenous zones. Rather, he will test your desire and, approaching you step by step, respond to your

permission. He'll also be expecting your response while he ca-resses you, sensing your most satisfying spots based on your re-actions. These are the most astute men and the ones who will really help you enjoy the experience.

7. Don't be fooled by physical attraction, and don't be impressed by men who boast of their sexual prowess. Consider men who have a more modern masculinity, who are less aggressive in making decisions and who are more appropriate for a satisfac-tory sexual relationship with you.

Advice for Men

1. There is a prototype of the subjugating, super-attractive woman who is a trap for unwary men. She seems to move around like a lioness looking for her mate, seduces with the way she talks, absent-mindedly moves her legs or skirt, and is playfully provocative. Distrust her if she is watching you while openly showing that she desires you. This is a warning that you are "jumping into the abyss again." Surely you'll have good sex, but afterward you'll flee through the first door you can find. Once again, you'll feel empty and will ask yourself: Do I really have to be a superman?

2. Ask yourself: Whom do I have to satisfy? Maybe you have asked yourself this question previously. Even if myths and petty talk tell you otherwise, after the first time a man does need to feel protected. He needs to be sure that his mate had a good time and that he made her enjoy the sex act.

3. Surely you don't want to simply add one more orgasm to your score. That is why you should attentively observe this woman you have in front of you. Smell her fragrance and caress her

skin delicately until you feel you both can be one single body. If you're not sure, learn to wait for a more appropriate time.

4. Take as long as you need. No one is going to think you're not manly enough. This is only a test for your own satisfaction and sometimes it is worth it to wait a little longer.

26

USING FRAGRANCES AND MASSAGE TO ENHANCE PLEASURE

Fragrances to Delight Yourself and Others

For the ancient Greeks, daily aromatic baths combined with massage opened the way to total sexual actualization. Nowadays, sensual aromatherapy has again become one of the most effective techniques to revitalize passion in marital life.

Many ancient arts that were discarded for centuries by institutional medicine indeed contain a great deal of truth in their aim to improve personal well-being and practice the art of loving to the fullest.

Oils, Fragrances, and Other Delights

The aromatherapy that is currently the rage among the restless generations of our youth is a healing procedure performed by inhaling different aromas. But direct aspiration through the nose is only one of the basic methods to administer the essential oils, perfumes, and salts.

They can also be applied to the skin in the course of immersion baths and erotic or relaxing massages, as well as in warm packs applied to the erogenous zones of the body. Aromatherapy is advisable for those couples who are starting an emotional and sexual relationship, because it helps them overcome more quickly the lack of mutual trust they experience at first.

In this case, if the massage is started at the soles of the feet, the essential oils will be absorbed more quickly and their stimulating effects will generate a greater sense of relaxation and sexual attraction.

An Erotic Massage Technique to Perform as a Couple

Erotic massages can be performed with different types of oils that stimulate the circulation of blood and sexual desire. In men, the technique will be most effective if applied to the area of the testicles. In women, this will be achieved by finding her most sensitive spots while caressing her under the influence of these fragrances.

Pure essential oils are obtained from the bark, roots, stems, leaves, flowers, and resins of plants and trees. To inhale their intoxicating aromas, place the essence of your choice in a pressure cooker. The steam will spread the perfume throughout the house and create a delightful environment. The fragrance may also be burned in a special container.

Magical Love Recipes: How to Prepare Homemade Essential Oils

In ancient times, plants and flowers were pressed and then infusions were prepared until the process of distillation was perfected. Presently, you can make a perfume with the plant of your choice by placing it in water and allowing the surplus water to evaporate. Allow the product to cool, and the essential oil will separate from the water. You can use flower petals, fruit rinds, and all kinds of plants with their multiple potentials.

The Purpose of Each Aroma

There are numerous books that explain aromatherapy in plain language. In those books we can find descriptions of the various methods of using fragrances along with specific recommendations. The brief list given here only mentions a few of the aromas that can accompany and enhance love. Fragrances affect everyone differently, so it is up to each couple to find out which aromas facilitate ecstasy for them.

Orange Blossom

A sedative, relaxing. Predisposes you to a dreamlike state.

Bergamot

Acts against negative thoughts. Reduces fears and calms anxiety.

Cinnamon

A special aphrodisiac for those with a lack of sexual desire.

Cedar

Stimulating. A mild aphrodisiac. Calms anxiety. Lifts the spirit and purifies the mind.

Mint

A tonic and stimulant for sexual desire.

Jasmine

A powerful healing agent for emotional disorders. Elevates the mood and stimulates erection.

Lemon

A natural energy-inducing tonic. Helps reduce inflammation of the erogenous zones.

Orange

Strengthens the heart and improves the body.

Patchouli

Comes from a small plant that is native to Malaysia and India, with a sedative and aphrodisiac effect. It may be used in the form of incense to calm excessive anxiety toward the sexual response.

Rosemary

Both the Greeks and Romans believed that rosemary was a sacred plant with magical powers. It is a stimulant for the glands and respiratory airways and therefore increases the energy of the sexual rhythm.

Rose

Arabic physicians were the first to use roses as medication in the form of *zuccar,* i.e., rose marmalade. This essence regulates the functioning of the female sexual organs. It acts as an aphrodisiac, an antidepressant, a sedative, and a tonic for the heart, stomach, liver, and uterus.

27

APHRODISIACS: PLEASURE FOODS

Aphrodisiacs: Foods to Enhance Enjoyment

There are foods that awaken the senses, increase circulation and sexual potency, and enhance vital instincts. If you get to know them, you'll be able to enjoy your lover more after a perfect meal.

The Origins of Aphrodisiacs

The first historical references on the stimulating effects of certain vegetables on sexual appetite date back to the most ancient writings. Since the beginning of history, humans have looked for magical foods to seduce their mates, and in that search they have found the right ingredients. But humans have also tried to find the source of eternal pleasure, the magical substance that will give them the ability, desire, and potency to prolong their sexual intimacy.

In all cultures and times, experiencing the utmost pleasure has been one of the human objectives. Prolongation, enjoyment, and permanent innovation have caused humans to insistently seek thousand of formulas to heighten desire. Previously, it was believed that all food arriving from exotic places contained magical erotic properties. That's why the discovery of America and its various unknown crops became the rage in European courts.

The idea of romantic love stimulated by extraneous substances, used to perform all kinds of erotic feats, became the fashion during the Renaissance. Asparagus and carrots, because of their phallic shape, were commonly used and famous at that time.

Observations back then were primitive and confused magical rituals with empirical observations. For example, if the root of a plant resembled the genitals, that plant was considered to have an aphrodisiac effect.

Oriental Rites

In Japan, an aphrodisiac meal does not consist simply of the foods ingested. Tradition emphasizes the use of the *tatami,* the place of the ceremony, where people must come in barefoot in order to leave behind the negative spirits that may have remained stuck to the soles of their shoes.

Observing the precept of ceremonial cleanliness, participants wipe their hands and faces with a wet towel. The meals that are then ingested are based on various seafoods. However, in order for them to really have an aphrodisiac effect, the whole environment must be charged with eroticism, as must the lovers' attitude.

Aphrodisiac Foods

The following foods generate higher levels of erotic energy. However, remember that the true food is love, and love keeps longer and better than any aphrodisiac, stimulating all the cells of the body and keeping the spirit forever young. Sexual pleasure is unlimited for those who liberate their minds through the true knowledge of all of their sexual powers.

Angelfish

This fish has an exquisite taste. Its use dates back to the Middle Ages. It is cooked just like the stingray.

Apples

In ancient times, if a woman shared an apple with a man, it was considered to be a token for a future betrothal.

Basil

"Woman is like a fruit that won't surrender its sweetness until you press it with your hands. Look at basil: if you don't press on it with the warmth of your fingers, it will not yield any perfume" (Sheik Nefzawi). This plant was consecrated to Venus, and in India to Vishnu.

Bee Pollen

Bee pollen increases virility and prolongs life.

Cacao

Cacao seeds contain phenylethylamine, a natural stimulant of the body. The Aztecs considered cacao a food for the gods.

Cardamom

Cardamom seeds enjoy high regard in Oriental cuisine and are an ingredient in curry. The Kama Sutra offers this aphrodisiac recipe: Mix cardamom with ginger and cinnamon. Spread it over onions and peas.

Celery

Celery contains pheromones. It may be drunk as a tea, or eaten in salads, soups, and stews.

Cinnamon

The second bark of the cinnamon tree, with a yellowish-red color, is very pleasant and aromatic. It is used particularly in desserts, but also in soups and stews. It's an aphrodisiac, an antiseptic, an astringent, and a stimulant.

Clams

Many cultures, like the American culture, blindly believe that clams have aphrodisiac properties, a belief that is indeed true, especially if they're eaten raw.

Clove

Clove is used as a spice. It is a powerful ingredient in some aphrodisiac potions.

Cockles

Cockles can be eaten both raw and cooked.

Coriander

The very aromatic and pleasant-tasting coriander seeds are ground and then used in love potions.

Endive

Endive clears the body of its impurities and has an invigorating and tonic effect.

Figs

The Greeks and Romans considered figs to be aphrodisiacs.

Garlic

The recognition enjoyed by garlic as an aphrodisiac tonic probably originated from its noticeable heating effect on the body. Current research shows that it reduces blood pressure and fat levels. It enhances vitality and health, which are indispensable ingredients to render top sexual performance.

Ginger

The early peeled root of ginger stimulates circulation.

Ginseng

Ginseng is called the "cure all." Almost all properties have been attributed to it, some of them contradictory, such as being both a sedative and a stimulant. It is a general tonic and is also considered to increase sexual potency.

Guaraná

Guaraná is a climbing shrub spread throughout Brazil. Its hard seeds are used.

Herring

Herring is a powerful aphrodisiac according to Celtic culture. In addition to being a stimulant, it is also a marvelous revitalizer.

Jasmine

The exquisite, intoxicating perfume of jasmine fills the evening air in tropical climates.

Juniper

According to the Kama Sutra, tea made with juniper berries is a drink used to improve sexual vigor. It is not recommended for pregnant women and for anyone suffering from liver failure.

Mackerel

Mackerel is a fish with red meat and is not too popular. Smoked mackerel in hors d'oeuvres is a powerful aphrodisiac due to its quick effect.

Oysters

Considered to be one of the best aphrodisiacs, the powers of oysters are intensified if eaten raw.

Pepper

Black and white pepper come from the same berry, but white pepper doesn't contain the husk. Pepper is a stimulant and a muscle toner.

Plums

Plums are energy enhancers. They were administered in Elizabethan brothels.

Saffron

Saffron was used as an aphrodisiac by the Assyrians, Greeks, Phoenicians, and Arabs. It is said to stimulate the uterus and circulation.

Salmon

As an aphrodisiac, salmon is more potent than beef, and its effects are quicker.

Star Anise

With a taste similar to licorice, star anise should be used in moderation both in drinks and in foods.

Trout

Trout has the same properties as salmon.

Truffles

Truffles also contain pheromones, which is why they are considered an aphrodisiac.

Vanilla

Vanilla is a milder aphrodisiac.

Vervain

In ancient times, it was said that if you wanted to win a person's heart, all you had to do was rub your hands with vervain sap and touch that person.

Scallops

Scallops are one of the most powerful aphrodisiacs, second only to oysters.

Vitamin E

This vitamin has a marvelous effect on one's sexual life.

28

BODY ZONES AND HOW TO STIMULATE THEIR ENERGY WITH YOUR HANDS

Touch Heaven with Your Hands

Each area of your lover's body
is the reflection of your need to love him.
When your fingers slide down his figure,
you'll be able to read his wishes without looking.

Acupressure is the ancient technique of applying massages and subtle pressure along the energy meridians of the body. Its function is to release energy that is blocked by emotional or physical problems, which may lead to sexual or emotional dissatisfaction. The most frequent problems in men are impotence and premature ejaculation, and in women are frigidity and anorgasmy.

Acupressure is performed with the hands. It consists of massaging, pressing, and rubbing the area that must be stimulated. Thus we manage to relax the parts of the body that are under stress. As learning progresses, you'll find out which erogenous zones your partner needs you to stimulate in order to maintain a full and satisfying sexual relationship.

It is important to keep in mind that massages must be sensuously performed, so that your beloved does not perceive your moves as an invasion of his or her body. The sensation must be totally pleasant. When stress is evident, but your lover denies being tense or blocked, it is important to perform the massage in a very subtle fashion. To the extent that intimacy progresses in the relationship, your mate will accept your finger stimulation.

Magic Fingers, Effective Massages

It is essential to practice this massage technique on a permanent basis. Lovers can take about ten minutes to explore their partner's body before the sex act.

Relax before you start in order to release all your daily worries.

Once you finish the relaxation, slide your hands down your lover's body with soft caresses, using any relaxing or toning oil.

Connect with your partner through your hands and through your eyes, speaking affectionate words that enhance the relationship.

Synchronize your breathing, especially if you are massaging each other, so that your circulatory rhythms function as one.

Start the massage at the soles of your partner's feet and, slowly, press slightly on the sides of the legs, advancing along the midline of the legs with ascending motions.

In men, light rubbing should be performed up the legs, through the hips, and then up to the area of the pelvis. If possible, use essential oils on the testicles. This has an activating effect, but must be performed very softly. In women, the clitoris and the labia of the vagina should be massaged. Finger stimulation must be soft but direct.

The hands must work like energy radars, alert to the sensation of pleasure expressed by your mate at each movement. When your partner shows signs of fulfillment, it is important to keep focusing on that part of the body. That particular spot ought to be touched as often as possible at each new sexual contact.

Let your fingers move up over the belly and the area of the groin. Massage the body from side to side in the shape of a spiral until you reach the pectoral muscles. This area is highly erotic for women and for men. Continue surrounding the pectoral area in circles, around the nipple, until you finally stimulate it directly.

If at this stage of the massage the sexual games have not started, you can continue acupressure by following the line of the spine, with light pressure on the ending point of each vertebra until you reach the neck.

Activate the ear area with light rubbing, because our organs are reflected in this site, from inside out. Finish with a light head massage to tone the scalp.

If you practice acupressure with the aim of perfecting the art of loving, you'll be able to assess the results with each sexual act. Its effectiveness will also be revealed in the growing strength of the couple's love bond in other important areas of their lives.

Sensual Massage for Couples

A sensual massage as a means to surprise and please your mate starts with a thorough preparation of the session and its environment, with the proper oils, controlled lighting, music for the occasion, and selection of the ideal moment. To this we must add imagination and devoted care. When the hands talk as they move over the body, the results can be unforgettable.

The preparation for a sensual and relaxing massage session can in itself be a complete experience for the senses. Attention and meticulous care play a major role in the final result—that is why we must be imaginative with respect to the environment we wish to create.

We must choose the ideal moment for both partners and turn the location we have selected into a sensual space. Light, temperature, and music are essential, though we must not forget other complements, such as aromatic oils.

There are several kinds of oils. It is important to find the most pleasant one on the basis of its texture and aroma. If you desire to achieve an intense and effective sensual excitement, try using oils that are known for their aphrodisiac properties. Sandalwood, for instance, is an Oriental essence, with a woody scent and sedative effect. Patchouli, a more stimulating fragrance, has a sweet-smelling, mysterious smell. Or use ylang-ylang to provide a euphoric, sweet, and flowery perfume.

Before massaging your mate, you must first be very relaxed. You should not massage your partner if you're tired. Intimate contact in a couple is so close that even the deepest feelings are conveyed. The ideal thing is for both to relax and practice deep breathing in order to open up their minds and bodies, before beginning the massage.

It is important for the person who performs the massage to clear his or her mind and concentrate on the massage. Slow breathing, allowing your muscles to relax, will enhance your inner balance. Before you start massaging, you can ask your partner to softly massage your shoulders first. That way you have already received something before you start to give.

Symbiosis

Massaging is synonymous with touching, and touching in turn involves communication. The way a massage is given transmits the very feelings of the person who is giving it. It's as if a communication channel were opened whereby the person giving the massage is talking and the person receiving it is responding with his or her body.

The three basic types of manipulation are soft rubbing, kneading, and friction.

Soft Rubbing

Oil is applied in this type of rubbing to help you get to know your lover's body. You place your hands flat on your mate's back with your fingers relaxed and softly slide them down, trying to locate potential tension nodes. Pressure should usually be increased as your hands near the area of the heart. This has a relaxing effect, which is felt at the nerves located under the skin.

Kneading

Kneading consists of energetic motions that imitate the kneading of dough, and is particularly helpful for releasing accumulated tension. This type of manipulation is indicated for the more muscular regions. To do it well, you must press the skin between your thumb and your fingers and sink the thumb into the muscle mass. With your fingers, push the muscle toward you again. Move your hands, alternating between one and the other, pressing, pushing, and lifting the skin.

Friction

Friction consists of pressing rather small, specific areas, which induces a very pleasant, restful sensation. It is important to push the tip of the thumb downward and perform short rotational motions to achieve a deeper penetration. Friction has an analgesic effect and stimulates blood flow.

29

SEXUAL MAGIC

Introduction to Sexual Magic

Sexual magic leads to the union of body and soul. It transcends sex, space, and time. Sexual magic allows us to eliminate the negative aspects of a love relationship. It brings about a full enjoyment of life and a state of ecstasy that expands beyond the limits of our bodies until it achieves harmony with the universe.

When we speak of sexual magic, the reader usually associates it with casting "love spells" or, in the worst cases, using exotic recipes and secretly placing them in the food of some victim we want to win over. Some people may compare sexual magic with the degree of hypnosis or suggestion exerted by Count Dracula on the innocent Lucy.

In reality, sexual magic is the metaphysical explanation of how energy forces interact in a sexual relationship. They are the energies that attract and repel each other in the game of love.

When we talk about male or female energies as necessary elements for every sexual act, it is important to understand that female energy does not belong exclusively to women, nor does male energy belong exclusively to men. Both are part of our system. We all have them regardless of our gender.

Why does attraction take place between two bodies? The exchange of hormones is not the only thing that produces a pleasurable sexual contact. In a sexual act, both feelings and mental energy exert their influence. According to the magic ritual, a state of meditation before sex clears away the emotions that might have blocked the relationship. The mind becomes a sexual organ and contributes to the optimum workings of sexual magic.

The magical techniques used to get rid of negative thoughts and emotions are performed before and during intercourse. Sexual magic is not an action we mechanically perform, but rather a conscious exploration of our sexual and spiritual potential.

In order to implement these techniques, we must learn to eliminate fear. Ignorance of the limits of our sexual potential can provoke negative fantasies in a person or in the bond that binds a couple. We need to develop the feminine and masculine aspects of our inner selves. Each person, individually or with a partner, can attain an ever higher degree of ecstasy, which can reach an explosive state.

How to Practice Sexual Magic

If you do the exercise as a couple, it will be unforgettable for both of you. The lovers should sit down in front of each other and look at each other with the same trust and intimacy they experience when they look in a mirror, with the same attitude as when they see their own face in the morning.

Observe the other person without prejudice, as if that other person were a part of you and different only in appearance. If you are both undressed in a quiet place, the experience is much more powerful. If you start to feel the need to touch each other, that is because you are still avoiding the deep look I'm proposing. Observation must be, each time, ever more innocent. Try to get rid of sexual bodily perceptions and any emotions that may arise. Try to feel that way until you feel the other person as being a part of yourself.

If you do this by yourself, sit down in front of the mirror and perform the exercise the same way. It's possible that looking at your own body may also produce excitation. That's okay, because it shows that your vital energy is acting in a natural way. Don't repress your feelings—just observe without making any movement.

When you both feel that your minds are empty of the compulsion to act, then you can start to approach each other. At that moment, close your eyes.

Now listen to your hearts with your eyes closed. Without taking your own pulse, each of you should try to listen to the beating of your own heart, breathing and relaxing each time you release air. Become aware of the state of your body and try to perceive your partner's body intuitively without opening your eyes. This task is called *centering* and is an exercise that precedes magical meditation.

The centering state is essential, and it is also very easy to achieve. The objective is to train the body to be able to focus the mind wherever the will chooses. To do this, you both must learn to be present and relaxed and to get rid of the emotions that block sexual performance.

If you don't achieve centering after twenty minutes, you can still attain an optimum state by repeating the following affirmation mentally: "My relaxation is complete for the enjoyment of the spirit."

Magical Meditation:
The Path to Sexual Ecstasy

"A man and a woman . . .
The man is the eagle that flies.
The woman is the nightingale that sings.
To fly is to master space.
To sing is to conquer the soul.
The man is a temple.
The woman is the altar.
Before the temple we uncover ourselves;
before the altar we kneel down . . .
The man is where the Earth ends.
The woman is where Heaven starts."

—*Victor Hugo*

Relaxation exercises are part of the sexual magic technique. The first step is to concentrate before meditating, either individually or as a couple, to achieve mental and emotional control before having sex.

Prior to learning the next steps of this technique, we have to ask ourselves: How can we manage to concentrate on something so perfect as divinity if at the same time our whole body is excited and we feel the need to touch our partner?

The answer is not easy because, for thousands of years, men and women dutifully denied their sexuality and underestimated the energy of the sex act. But it is not that complicated either—you just need to feel a deep love for your partner and a great need to explore your sexual power beyond the limits of your imagination.

The act of learning to meditate ought to hold the same attraction for us as, for example, making love for the first time. It is an endearing, spiritual, and loving adventure, but the most important thing is to know that once one has been initiated in this technique, it is impossible to go back to the original state.

Now find a private place where you continue to follow all of the previous steps. Once you achieve this relaxed state, you should then center on your breathing. With each inhalation you must count to three, withhold the air, and exhale slowly. Your breathing must be almost imperceptible.

Once you achieve this state, locate in the area of your heart the most perfect and ideal image of what you wish to attain with your partner. If you can't visualize it, recreate internally a feeling or sensation that you would like to experience, without any prejudices. You should not see the image outside of you, as if it were projected onto a screen, but rather very vividly and with the full sensation of immediate experience.

After completing this concentration and creative visualization, you can take a few minutes to comment on the experience with your partner, without making comparisons.

If you performed the exercise individually, you can write about each visualization, as well as how the clarity, power, and strength of your meditation is evolving.

The success of this meditation can be observed when you experience greater control, confidence, and, above all, a feeling of happiness, in all aspects of your life.

The Keys to Opening and Developing Sexual Magic

To magically create our own universe, we need magical elements, such as light, space, time, and the channel for divine action—the human being. But the most important thing is not to forget that all human beings are equal or similar to our divine creator. This is the basis for the magic. Here are the keys to sexual magic.

Space

With your partner, look within your home for a place that is reasonably quiet. It does not have to be your bedroom. Any place where you know no one is going to bother you will do. Once there, get rid of all possible interferences, from the telephone to the television. Try to ventilate the environment and spread a soft aroma by burning myrrh or sandalwood incense. Turn off the lights. If possible, lightly illuminate the environment with a red candle.

Centering Yourself

Once you have succeeded in becoming centered, both of you should undress, which is also the best thing to do to get rid of your bodily inhibitions.

Perform the Protection Ritual

The first magical exercise you can try is a simple protection ritual. All you have to do is visualize a circle of light around your head that gradually descends throughout your body. The color of the energy with which you should meditate is brilliant white. Then imagine that same circle around yourself and around your partner's body. If you are by yourself, you can imagine it the same way, but you must feel as if your partner were present, sitting in front of you. Then you can expand the circle and surround the whole place, and then the whole house, until it finally surrounds the whole planet with its brilliant white light.

Focusing and Deepening

Try to focus mentally on the idea that this circle is protecting you and that nothing can happen to you, that the world is in harmony and complete fulfillment. Try to feel the ecstasy inside you, the peace and security of a world illuminated by a white light. If you still experience difficulties visualizing, try to think as if you were "daydreaming," but under your conscious control. It's like being reasonably attentive to what goes on around you, and still continuing to dream of your lover or partner or the whole universe surrounded by beauty and love.

With time and practice, you will be able to visualize anything you desire. You'll be able to practice a meditation that is more easily controlled each time, but it is not necessary for you to achieve this at the beginning. Try to maintain the state of ecstasy, control your breathing, and assess your state of relaxation on a permanent basis.

Erogenous Points

Now that you feel more relaxed, try to center on your heart, imagining that your mate is lying down. Visualize your partner and yourself as if you both were the God or Goddess of Love, and with this incomparable sensation imagine yourself caressing your lover's body. Think intuitively about the places where this person can feel the most pleasure. Don't get ahead of yourself—only caress your partner in your imagination. Don't focus on the parts of your lover's body that you like, but rather on those that you know are most pleasurable to your partner.

Intensification

With your eyes still closed, ask yourself: What is the level of intensity that I need in order to excite my lover? How far do I have to go in my exploration? What force or pressure do I have to exert?

Try to feel the ecstasy of the other person, and vibrate inside your mate's body as if it were your own.

Don't lose your concentration.

Don't open your eyes.

Don't lose your level of relaxation.

Continue performing this meditation until ecstasy becomes completely explosive.

30

RELATIONSHIPS WITH LOVE

The Seven Golden Rules

Our thoughts are creative—they create everything around us, especially everything that we focus on and comprehend. Sometimes our thoughts do this consciously and sometimes, in most cases, unconsciously. So if we want to change the world around us and our relationships, we have to start with our thoughts:

1. Our thoughts have the power to transform.
2. You are and have what you think and believe.
3. We have many thoughts per second; we need to make them conscious.
4. We can change everything we think.
5. We must be attentive to what we wish for and think . . .
6. . . . . to master our thoughts and not allow them to control us.

7. We have to exercise our thoughts daily—we need time and space to focus our energy to transform, to learn, and to evolve.

Creative Visualization Techniques

If we observe and investigate our internal world, we'll discover to what point our thinking is creative and powerful. To attain this excellent creative visualization, there are two steps that must be followed:

First Step: Complete Breathing

Complete breathing consists of working with the lungs and the abdomen to achieve a proper deep respiration. You must be lying down on the floor in a comfortable place where you won't be interrupted for about fifteen to thirty minutes.

At the beginning, until your breathing is natural and fluid, it is advisable to perform this exercise with your body at rest.

Pay attention to your thoughts and let them pass on as if they were a shower of energy—don't identify with any of them. After a few minutes of relaxation, place one hand on your abdomen and the other one on your chest. Let out all the air softly through your nose, emptying your lungs completely. Try to keep your lungs empty for a few seconds. Inhale slowly, inflating only your abdomen until you fill up the lower part of your lungs—without exerting yourself, you'll feel how your diaphragm expands downward. At this moment, the lower and middle parts of your lungs are full of air.

Before exhaling, take advantage of this moment and empty your mind of all your thoughts and imagine that you're also getting rid of all your daily tensions and emotions. Then move the air to the upper area of your lungs and, little by little, let it out.

Repeat this process for a minimum of ten minutes.

Second Step: Mental Concentration and Creative Visualization

Before starting the visualization exercise, have everything written down in detail so you have a clear view of what you want to achieve. You should clearly define each affirmation that you want to come true. For example:

1. Improve communication with your partner during dinner.
2. Understand your children better during the month of June.
3. Not have any problems at work today.

Let's consider the first example:

Visualize your partner and you sitting at home for dinner. When you do the exercise, don't imagine that you're watching a movie in your mind—try to feel, with all your senses, what you're visualizing as if you were really doing it.

Then imagine a scene in which there is little communication between the two of you, and scratch out that mental image with a huge X. Add to this imaginary action the word *canceled*.

Then imagine you both having a friendly and affectionate dinner, with all the details you want included. Ideally you should do two creative visualizations a day until they come true. Once a visualization has become real, keep working on new ones, but never visualize more than two images a day.

The mind is very literal and orderly. Always remember that if we have the capacity to dream, it is because we also have the ability to make those dreams come true.

Relationships with Love

Creating relationships with love is to participate in the celebration of love that the universe offers each day. We have inside ourselves a dark corner that keeps us from enjoying life. We can illuminate this corner with mental clarity and a willing heart. Life is a beautiful invitation. Do you want to enjoy all aspects of love? Don't procrastinate. It all depends on you.

The Path Toward a Mind of Light

Visualization enables you to have a harmonious relationship with your own self and with others. It consists of four steps:

Clearing the Mind

The purpose of clearing the mind is to quiet the roaring stream of thoughts that flows all the time. This objective is achieved through good, full breathing.

Observing the Mind

For visualization to be effective, you must be attentive to the thoughts that crop up in your mind. When you lose your concentration, relax again and pay attention to your breathing. A very interesting meditation involves realizing how the chain of thoughts operates, how thoughts are linked to each other.

Disciplining the Mind

In this step we have to penetrate the contents of thought, and see how one thought leads to another and then on to another and how they are all linked. You don't have to get involved with these thoughts; just observe how the process takes place without paying too much attention to what the actual subject of thought is, because oftentimes it is emotional energy that finds its way to the mental plane.

Affirmations

Discipline enables the mind to use affirmations. Affirmations are one of the most powerful tools at the mind's disposal, and are achieved by fixing the affirmation and visualizing it clearly. An affirmation can also be repeated like a mantra. Ideally, each affirmation should be repeated fifteen minutes a day until it comes true.

The Different Kinds of Relationships and Emotional Energy

The world is full of positive and negative energy. Emotions are one aspect of it. There is a separation between emotions that are incorrectly called negative and emotions that are incorrectly called positive. Emotions are simply energies in motion. What makes them positive or negative is what we do with them and the effects they have on our relationships. Anger, hate, and fear are emotions that are called negative because they block us, make us ill, and torment us. Love, hope, and affection are called positive because they heal us, give us relief, and protect us. All emotions are part of life, but how can we manage our emotions?

Learning to Have Relationships with Love

To be able to love, we have to control our fears and the negative energy they produce. The following steps help create a good internal basis:

1. The mind cannot entertain two thoughts at the same time; therefore, when the first negative thought comes up, clear your mind and cancel that thought. You will discipline your mind and learn to focus on the positive.

2. Try to discover the source of each negative emotion that crops up. This will lead you to self-knowledge and wisdom.

3. Avoid judging or censuring others. It is better to try to reinforce and strengthen the positive we see in others; otherwise, the finger you point at them tomorrow may be pointed back at you. If you strive to see the good both in you and others, very soon you'll be much happier.

4. Living in darkness is not the same as remaining in a dark chamber—it means not being able to see the reality of life in harmony and light. You may choose to live always in darkness, but if you tire of it, you can turn on the light. Seeing clearly is a mental exercise that is achieved by gaining an awareness of all your positive emotions until you discover the best in you.

5. Observe role models or attitudes that you would like to imitate. Having a positive role model can be of help, provided you don't idealize that person.

6. Choose which emotions you want for your relationships. You should have control over your life and your emotions. Try to observe each stimulus that comes to you, how you react, and what effect it produces in you. This mechanism will provide you with permanent self-awareness.

7. Bring to mind all opportunities open to you. When you believe you're hurt by the effect of your negative emotions, make a list of all the positive ways in which you could respond to this situation. This system creates a protective mechanism that will never fail you.

8. Visualize this list and work on the daily affirmations until you achieve your goal.

Remember how many times you have lost your footing while you were on the path of insecurity and fear. Now is the time to tread along the path of love. Your perfect guide will be the sweet whisperings that always spring from your heart.

31

FREEDOM: THE GIFT OF LOVE

Sexual Freedom: The Path to Truth

Sexual freedom is a slogan so trite and oversold that most of us have lost sight of what it really means. Freedom is a natural gift that depends on each human being's knowledge, clarity of mind, and internal development.

You are free when there is coherence between your inner world and the external universe. This is expressed when you give and receive the best in you naturally and spontaneously—when you enjoy each experience as a game of energies that flow incessantly, and enjoy the present without expecting to receive the approval of others. You trust and follow the dictates of your own heart.

To maintain an active and free sexual life, we must respect the same principles.

1. Know your inner world.
2. You are and have what you think and believe.

3. Become more aware of your powers and limitations.

4. Keep your feelings, beliefs, thoughts, and actions mutually consistent.

5. Enjoy each moment and each erotic encounter, aware that it is a unique and unrepeatable moment of pleasure with your partner.

6. Seek the satisfaction of your partner in a natural and fluid way.

7. Be open to receive, while giving emotional and sexual satisfaction at each encounter.

However . . . how can you really practice all of these universal principles? What is the guidance you need? Beyond sex, color, religion, or social status, there are keys to maintaining the balance in the scales:

1. Love and protect your own body.

2. Know the whole body as a pleasure map for your own satisfaction and for that of your partner.

3. Trust the body language in the erotic encounter.

4. Be attentive and open to all the signals your mate gives you in a sexual relationship.

5. Understand, nonjudgmentally, the sexual fantasies that issue from your mind.

6. Respect the desires, beliefs, and ideas of others.

7. Be open to enjoying new experiences proposed by your partner, while remaining true to your own needs.

8. Look for and update information on new techniques to enhance pleasure.

9. Understand that erotic contact is a fascinating game and exchange between two people.

10. Take care of the health of your body and the body of your lover, protecting it from any disease.

11. Maintain a sexual ethic with your partner, which entails respecting his or her availability and the codes agreed to for each new encounter.

12. Remember your erotic dreams to try to find their unconscious messages and understand the hidden meaning being expressed.

13. Try to observe any resistance to feeling when you're with your partner.

14. Always propose sexual communication without imposing rules that are not shared by your partner.

15. Respect other people's sexual tendencies, which does not imply participating in them.

16. Try to get information on, and clarify everything related to, the myths that condition our sexuality.

17. Maintain a renewed attitude on the erotic plane, regardless of how long you have been in the relationship.

18. Seek open spaces in which full harmony can flourish.

The liberation of a human being, in all areas of his or her life, and in different forms, is endowed with an infinite essence. The wisdom of enjoying life in full freedom consists of discovering each day a new aspect of love.

32

FORMULAS FOR TENDERNESS

If you can't remember the last time someone waited for you with open arms, open your book and jot down a few tricks to prevent the decline and decay of your life as a couple.

Go over just the past few weeks: How many times did you wish for the person you love to take you in his or her arms by surprise? How many other times have you felt overwhelmed by an absence of tenderness in your relationship? Do you feel you have lost forever the passion of the first glorious days with your lover? Could you experience again, with the same enthusiasm, those fleeting summer loves, brimming with ardent fantasies? How long can you suffer from a lack of fulfillment before you start to beg for a little affection due to the lack of tenderness in your daily life?

You need to have a few ingredients handy that will improve the nature of each encounter:

Don't Keep Track of Complaints

If you wish to have a more pleasant relationship, avoid misunderstandings and exhausting arguments.

Laughter

The ability to laugh at yourself and find something positive in difficult situations holds a great deal of potential tenderness.

Silence

Learn to value your partner's need for silence when he or she needs to feel you or simply to observe you. These are moments brimming with tenderness.

Surprise

Routine is the worst enemy of affection. A couple can transform this state of inertia only if they learn to think of those small but eternal details that bring happiness to their life together. Discovering how to keep tenderness alive is an incredible game with thousands of creative combinations. In your agenda, prepare a list of surprises for your beloved.

Timing

The most difficult aspect of a love relationship is knowing how to find the right moment to discuss the things that bother us, irritate us, and hamper pleasure.

Generosity

Generosity means having the intention of giving without expecting to receive an expression of love or sexual desire from your partner.

Other Ideas

Other ingredients to promote tenderness in a relationship include respect, tactfulness, understanding, and especially the willingness to propose new or different ideas to foster a more positive relationship. Be alert to what the other person wants to express. Words don't always express what we really feel. Oftentimes emotions that are deep find a good hideaway in and behind our words.

Being willing to love and relax, and devote ourselves in body and soul to our partner is not a dream or an old-fashioned illusion. Giving the other person (and ourselves) the opportunity to enjoy his or her share of true tenderness, even for an instant, also affords us an oasis in our daily struggle.

33

HOW TO FIND
YOUR SOUL MATE

How to Find the Love of Your Life

Your soul longs for another who has all the qualities that are in harmony with yours. But your senses confuse you and distract you from
your true love. By concentrating on your heart, you will be able to find
the love of your life. Now get ready to discover the power of love.

The Calling of the Heart

You may be in the presence of your true love and fail to notice that
person because your senses distract you from him or her. For example,
let's say you have to put away a very important object and for some reason suddenly become distracted from what you're doing (it could be a
phone call or something on the radio that catches your attention). You
do put away the object, but then forget where you placed it. You lose

the object that was so important to you because it slipped through your fingers, or you put it in a place that you can't remember.

Your existence can pass by in oblivion or in perfect harmony—it depends solely on you.

All meditation and creative visualization techniques are based on concentrating our thoughts on a point, object, situation, location, person, archetype, image, mantra, or desire. There is a basic principle that is the basis for all mental concentration theories: energy follows thought. This means that anything you think will always be sustained by a physical, emotional, mental, or spiritual energy from which the object of your desire will materialize. There is no doubt that whatever you truly desire in your heart will first become a reality in your inner world and then manifest itself on the external plane.

Commitment of the Divine Power to Create

Before implementing these techniques, you must become aware of the power of your will.

First, be aware and know that we are creators of the universe, because our thoughts create.

Second, you must be very honest with yourself before going ahead with your desire to find the love of your life. Try to answer the following questions:

Do I wish to find my one and final lover?

Do I have a clear idea of the lover I need?

Am I ready for the love of my life?

Do I wish to experience many relationships before having a full and true commitment to the love of my life?

Have I dreamed of the possibility of finding a harmonious and perfect relationship?

Am I willing to live this adventure?

Am I only interested in the external appearance of my lover or am I also interested in my partner's deeper qualities?

Finding the Divine Lover

For this technique to be truly effective, prior to the visualization exercise you must write down how you picture your perfect lover in as much detail as possible.

Remember that universal energy and thought are very literal and specific. An ancient proverb says: "Be careful what you wish for because it just may come true."

First Step

Concentrate on the essential attributes you wish to find in your special person.

Second Step

Mold and shape your lover—try to see your lover's interior clearly so that it may later be manifested on the outside. Structure the image as a reality that is in the here and now, in the present time.

Write affirmations that create the perfect lover. For example: "I found the person of my dreams. He/she always understands me and is able to help me. My mate is perfect, he/she always fills me. With my perfect lover, sexual relations bring me surprise, tenderness, and ecstasy. My lover is very beautiful and thinks I'm perfect for him/her."

Do not write the name of a specific person but rather let the law of attraction do its work, and trust universal energy.

Third Step

Perform full breathing when it becomes clear to you what you want to visualize.

Fourth Step

Visualize the perfect lover, following the affirmations you have created. The purpose of this technique is twofold: to awaken your inner capacity to love and to be able to recognize your lover in the external world.

Fifth Step

With your thoughts and feelings, and through daily visualization or meditation, you have to create your self-love platform. By doing this, each day you will become more convinced that you are indeed loved and unconditionally accepted in a way that is perfect for you.

In order for visualization to work, it is essential to have the inner certainty that you can bring out the best in yourself. The other major point is being alert and always having an open heart to receive the love of your life.

Twin Souls

The magnetic attraction between two kindred spirits is inevitable and, even though it is said that the ideal lover cannot always be found, this wonderful phenomenon is experienced at least once in the life of a person. In fact, the encounter usually happens way before the concrete discovery of that other person takes place.

It commonly happens that we have lived the experience without knowing, because affinity is usually so subtle that our ego may ignore the presence of that other part of our being.

Levels of Union of Souls

Each human being experiences this marvelous event on different planes of energy:

First Level

The first level of union is spiritual. This plane is reached when twin souls are internally ready to be united. Both parties feel a great sense of fulfillment, and, if the union is spiritual, it is possible that they will never be apart again.

Second Level

The second plane is intellectual: twin souls are in agreement on what they think.

Third Level

The third level is emotional. From the first encounter there is an intense affinity and the feeling of having known each other for a long time. During this stage, twin souls fall in love more easily. They share a great sense of surrender and equilibrium.

Fourth Level

The fourth level is physical or erotic. The partners in a couple consisting of twin souls surrender to each other physically and with boundless passion. In the sexual act, kisses and embraces are intense and endless because, in their physical contact, they feel that they have finally found their true home. On the erotic plane, twin souls discover from the first moment that their partner knows their body to perfection. They caress and kiss each other as if they were one single body, and their erotic encounters may succeed in reaching beyond space and time because both perceive that they are being transported to another dimension. The sensation of freedom and of flight while they make love is sublime, and they feel they can touch heaven with their hands.

Without this last physical level, twin souls cannot truly recognize themselves as a couple. If they relate on the other planes of unconditional love, their relationship may manifest as a long-lasting friendship, or as a special affection between two people, without merging as a couple. This will depend on the personality, the spiritual development, and the degree of self-awareness of each party.

How to Find Your Twin Soul

If the rational side of a person insists on ignoring the soul's desires, it's surely because that person has a mental message that is telling him or her: "It is impossible for someone like that to exist." Or: "All that stuff about twin souls is a well-meaning tale, but I'll never get to experience it."

What is true is that when you are ready for the encounter, you will attract the other person like a magnet, provided negative emotions or thoughts don't hamper this process. In order to live the thrilling experience of discovering a kindred spirit, you don't need to be a certain age. Where can you find that kindred spirit? It may be in school, college, work, on a trip, on the Internet, or under the most unexpected circumstances.

In love, there are no recipes or conditions, and there are no rules. To invoke your twin soul, you need to have a deep knowledge of your own self.

34

THE PERFECT LOVER
MAKES LOVE
WITH BODY AND SOUL

Trust Yourself

You are the soil where all things rest.
You are the earth whence all things spring forth.
You are here, you are solid, you are alive.
You are the point where all things
in the universe begin.

It has always been asserted that the most erotic zone of every human being starts and ends in oneself.

In Tantric philosophy, sex is the union between the earth and the universe—human beings act within this sexual union like a channel or bridge having an infinite and eternal erotic force.

Due to ignorance, the true function of sex has always been a mystery, particularly its origin or the root cause that generates such an excitement in every human being.

No one can deny that sexual energy is the most subtle and powerful energy in our existence. Vitality is directly related to sexuality, combining the three spheres of life: thought, feeling, and will.

The result of the various modifications of these three factors generates the most sensual and profound sexual desire, both in relation to oneself and to others.

If your attitude with respect to sex is not based on philosophical arguments or negative or positive prejudices, you will open up to the understanding of Tantra. Only in this way can eroticism be useful, because sexual energy is difficult to control, difficult to handle, difficult to know, and difficult to store. If we manage to be ever more conscious of our sexual impulses, we'll be able to live in paradise.

Our intuition will guide us to do the right thing. Conscious knowledge of what causes sexual desire is part of the training and the willingness to channel our vital forces in a truly beneficial way.

Making Love with the Universe

Tantra states:

"Accept yourself just as you are. You are a great mystery consisting of many energies that combine on many dimensions.

Accept this mystery and move with each energy, with deep sensitivity,

with clear-mindedness, with love, with understanding.

Then each desire will become a vehicle

for self-improvement.

Each energy will be an aid to you,

and the world itself conscious light in your life.

Your own body is a temple, a sacred place,

where the universe pays homage."

EPILOGUE

The Tao Plays No Favorites

The infinite Tao flows everywhere,
creating and destroying,
actualizing the world,
minding the smallest details,
Asking nothing in return.
It nourishes all things, without controlling them;
it lacks intention,
and therefore appears to be inconsistent.

It is the substance of all things,
but it doesn't subject or control anything;
it makes no exceptions,
that is why it is important to everything.
And because it does not favor any finite thing,
it is infinite.

—Tao Te King, 34

BIBLIOGRAPHY

Arnold, Paul. *Con los sabios místicos de Japón*. Buenos Aires:
   Editorial Dédalo, 1976.

Asín Cabrera, A. *Tantra*. Madrid: Editorial Analecta, 1980.

Ballesteros Arránz, Ernesto. *Yogasûtras de Patâñjali*. Madrid:
   Ediciones Bhisma, 1993.

Benson, Herbert, M.D. *Relajación*. Barcelona: Editorial Pomaire, 1977.
   Also published in English as *The Relaxation Response*.
   Avon, 1990.

Bernard, Jean-Luis. *El tantrismo, yoga sexual*. Barcelona: A. T. E., 1975.

Bernard, Theos. *El camino práctico del yoga: el cielo está
   en nosotros*. Buenos Aires: Editorial La Pléyade, 1972.

———. *Hatha yoga: una técnica de liberación*. Buenos Aires:
   Ediciones Siglo Veinte, 1973.

Besant, Annie. *El yoga*. Buenos Aires: Editorial Kier, 1966.

Calle, Ramiro. *La sabiduría de los grandes yoguis.* Barcelona: Círculo de Lectores, 1975.

——. *Principios de yogoterapia.* Madrid: Ediciones Pirámide, 1979.

——. *Yoga: ciencia de la salud.* Madrid: Ediciones Pirámide, 1979.

Chang, Jolan. *Tantra: el culto de lo femenino.* Sudamericana Grupo Editor.

Comunidad del Arco Iris. *Tantra, la alquimia energética, Volumen I.* Barcelona: Arcoiris, 1981.

Eliade, Mircea. *Yoga, inmortalidad y libertad.* Buenos Aires: Editorial La Pléyade, 1977.

Feuerstein, George. *The Philosophy of Classical Yoga.* Rochester: Inner Traditions International, 1996.

——. *The Shambhala Encyclopedia of Yoga.* Boston: Shambhala Publications, Inc., 1997.

——. *The Yoga Tradition: Its History, Literature, Philosophy and Practice.* Prescott: Hohm Press, 1998.

Guenon, René. *La metafísica oriental.* Barcelona: Ediciones de la Tradición Unánime, 1984.

Herrigel, Eugen. *Zen en el arte del tiro con arco.* Buenos Aires: Editorial Kier, 1979.

Holleman, Dona. *Dancing the Body of Light.* The Netherlands: Pegasus Enterprises, 1999.

Iam, Mabel. *El don de la diosa.* Buenos Aires: Editorial Mega Libros, 1999.

——. *Magia sexual.* Tienda de Libros, 2001.

Jung, Carl. *Arquetipos e inconciente colectivo.* Buenos Aires: Editorial Paidós, 1974.

——. *Contribución a los símbolos.* Buenos Aires: Editorial Paidós.

———. *Energética psíquica y esencia del sueño.* Buenos Aires: Editorial Paidós, 1982.

———. *Formaciones de lo inconciente.* Buenos Aires: Editorial Paidós.

———. *La interpretación de la naturaleza y la psique.* Buenos Aires: Editorial Paidós, 1994.

———. *La psicología de la transferencia.* Buenos Aires: Editorial Paidós.

———. *Las relaciones entre el yo y el inconciente.* Buenos Aires: Editorial Paidós.

———. *Lo inconciente.* Editorial Losada.

———. *Los complejos y el inconciente.* Editorial Alianza, 1970.

———. *Psicología y alquimia.* Buenos Aires: Editorial Paidós.

———. *Psicología y educación.* Buenos Aires: Editorial Paidós.

———. *Psicología y religión.* Buenos Aires: Editorial Paidós.

———. *Psicología y simbología del arquetipo.* Buenos Aires: Editorial Paidós.

———. *Realidad del alma.* Editorial Losada.

———. *Recuerdos, sueños y pensamientos.* Editorial Seix Barral S.A., 1966.

———. *Simbología del espíritu.* Fondo de Cultura Economica, 1962.

———. *Símbolos de transformación.* Buenos Aires: Editorial Paidós, 1982.

———. *Sincronicidad.* Buenos Aires: Editorial Paidós.

———. *Teoría del psicoanálisis.* Editorial Plaza y Janes.

———. *Tipos psicológicos.* Editorial Sudamericana.

Jung, Carl, y otros. *El hombre y sus símbolos.* Editorial Caralt.

Jung, Carl, y Wilhelm, R. *El secreto de la flor de oro.* Buenos Aires: Editorial Paidós, 1981.

Jung, Carl, Campbell, J., Bly, Keen, Dossey, May, Branden, Wilber, Hillman, Bradshaw. *Encuentro con la sombra.* Editorial Kairos.

Jung, Carl, Campbell, J., Harding, Zweig, Stein, Bly, Rich, Hillman, Von Franz, Whitmont, y otros. *Espejos del yo*. Editorial Kairós.

Krishnamurti. *El estado creativo de la mente*. Buenos Aires: Editorial Kier.

——. *La libertad primera y última*. Barcelona: Editorial Kairós, 1996.

Lao Tse. *Tao Te Ching*. Barcelona: Ediciones Orbis, 1985.

——. *Tao-Te-King*. Madrid: Luis Cárcamo, editor, 1980.

Lysebeth, Andre Van. *Tantra: el culto de lo femenino*. Barcelona: Ediciones Urano, 1990.

Osho. *Aquí y ahora*. Editorial Libros de Osho.

——. *De la medicación a la meditación*. Editorial Libros de Osho.

——. *Introducción al mundo del tantra*. Roselló Impressions.

——. *¿Qué es meditación?* Roselló Impresions.

——. *Sólo un cielo*. Roselló Impresions.

——. *Tao: los tres tesoros*. Editorial Libros de Osho.

——. *Tantra: espiritualidad y sexo*. Editorial Libros de Osho.

——. *Una nueva visión sobre la liberación de la mujer*. Editorial Gulaab.

——. *Vida, amor y risa*. Editorial Libros de Osho.

——. *Yoga: la ciencia del alma, volumen II*. Editorial Gulaab.

——. *Zen: tarot*. Editorial Libros de Osho.

Ramacharaka, Yogi. *14 lecciones sobre filosofía yogi y ocultismo oriental*. Buenos Aires: Editorial Kier, 1972.

——. *Ciencia hindú yogi de la respiración*. Buenos Aires: Editorial Kier, 1973.

Raynaud de la Ferriere, Serge. *Yug, yoga, yoguismo*. Mexico: Editorial Diana, 1975.

Reid, Daniel. *El tao de la salud, el sexo y la larga vida*. Barcelona: Editorial Urano, 1989. Also published in English as *Tao of Health, Sex & Longevity*. Redwing Book Co., 1999.

Rinpoché, Sogyal. *Meditación*. Editado por: José J. de Olañeta. Palma, 1998.

Riviere, Jean. *El yoga tántrico*. Buenos Aires: Editorial Kier, 1978.

Salzberg, Sharon. *Amor incondicional*. Madrid: Editorial Edaf, 1987.

Sama, Meishu. *Foundation of Paradise*. Johrei Fellowship.

———. *The Art of the Johrei*. Lux Oriens.

Shankara. *La joya suprema del discernimiento*. Edicomunicaciones.

Shankaracharya, Sri. *La joya suprema del discernimiento y la realización directa*. Buenos Aires: Editorial Kier.

Sing Khalsa, Gurudass. *Kundalini yoga, tal como lo enseña Yogui Bhajan*. Barcelona: Editorial Alas, 1989.

Sivananda, Kalyan. *Instituto tantra*. Buenos Aires: Editorial Kier, 1979.

Sivananda, Swami. *Ciencia del pranayama*. Buenos Aires: Editorial Kier, 1975.

———. *Kundalini Yoga*. Buenos Aires: Editorial Kier, 1971.

———. *Tantra Yoga, Nada Yoga, Kriya Yoga*. Buenos Aires: Editorial Kier, 1973.

Stoler Miller, Barbara. *Yoga: Discipline of Freedom: The Yoga Sutra Attributed to Patanjali*. Berkeley: University of California Press, 1996.

Suzuki y Fromm. *Budismo zen y psicoanálisis*. Madrid: Closas-Orcoyen, 1975.

Suzuki, D. T. *La práctica del monje zen*. Barcelona: Ediciones Abraxas, 1998.

Suzuki, Shunryu. *Mente zen, Mente de principiante*. Buenos Aires: Editorial Estaciones, 1987.

ABOUT THE AUTHOR

Mabel Iam is best known as a psychotherapist and expert in relationships, but she's also a favorite adviser to politicians and celebrities and the author of several award-winning, bestselling books around the world. She has rapidly become the number-one self-help expert in the United States.

Her books on sexuality, psychology, angels, and psycho-astrology are bestsellers in different countries and have earned her the Latino Literary Book Award for best self-help book, *Qué hay detrás de tu nombre,* granted by Latino Literacy Now at the 2003 Book Expo in Los Angeles. Besides, her books *Sex and the Perfect Lover* and *El Sueño del Amor* were nominated as best nonfiction books for the 2004 Latino Book Award by the Latino Literacy Now organization, at the NYC expo. The author has also received several awards for her career, among them the 1999 Mercosur Research Award.

Her career has picked up extraordinarily since the publication of *Sex and the Perfect Lover,* her first translation into English and her entrée into the Anglo-American market, which turned out to be such a success that the book was subsequently translated into Hungarian, Czech, French, German, and Portuguese, and was successfully sold in India. Her books have also been widely acclaimed by the press, in magazines like *Latina* and *Penthouse,* and in newspapers such as the *Miami Herald, El Diario La Prensa* (New York), *Journal, Críticas, Cosmopolitan TV,* and other newspapers in other languages.

Mabel has also reached millions of people in Argentina, her native country, and all over Latin America through her television and radio shows. Since 2002, she's been reaching out to TV viewers and radio listeners in the United States, where she now lives. She has a weekly column in *Radio Caracol* (Miami), and she writes for *El Diario−La Prensa* (New York) and participates in *Despierta América, Noticias 23,* and *De Mañanita,* on Univision and Telemundo, respectively.

From Miami, she continues to help millions of people through alchemy, psycho-astrology, Eastern Tao techniques, tantra, creative visualization, and angel invocation. Her work as an author and adviser has been published in prestigious international magazines and is disseminated in her seminars and workshops as well as at the main book expos in America.

In short, Mabel has always been on the cutting edge of self-help in Latin America and she is now ready to show off her full capacity and spiritual mastery all over the world.

Printed in the United States
By Bookmasters